Communication Skills
for Physiotherapists

D1344194

Communication Skills for Physiotherapists

VINCENT KORTLEVE MA (PSYCHOLOGY)

Physiotherapist
Viaperspectief
Driebergen, The Netherlands

ELSEVIER

ISBN: 978-0-7020-8398-3

Content Strategist: Robert Edwards
Content Project Manager: Shravan Kumar
Design: Julia Dummitt

Printed in Poland

Last digit is the print number: 9 8 7 6 5 4 3 2 1

Working together to grow libraries in developing countries

www.elsevier.com • www.bookaid.org

CONTENTS

by Stephen Rollnick

It is a privilege to write the foreword to this English translation of Vincent Kortleve's new book. I've often heard stories from friends about physiotherapists who made a difference in their lives, but I've also heard other stories that were not so positive. What makes the distinction? I think the great physiotherapists used communication and connection as a foundation for good practice, and the others did not. When I had my own experiences of being a patient and of running training workshops for physiotherapists in different countries, I was struck by two things: how well-rounded physiotherapists were in their manner and approach, and the healing potential they have in such intimate contact with their patients.

How can we champion the healing potential in physiotherapy consultations, knowing that the diversity of patient presentations is enough to keep the sharpest minds challenged? People come in with such a wide range of expectations, complaints, and concerns. One answer is in getting our communication right, and this is where Vincent Kortleve's new book stands out like a lighthouse. I have not come across another like it. It takes talent to write about experiences in everyday practice, and this book is based on many years of practice. It takes boldness to step across into other fields like motivational interviewing and to translate useful ideas into a form that will work well in practice. Here, again, Kortleve has done just that. Then there's the matter of keeping abreast of ongoing research and what comes out of efforts to understand the physiotherapy consultation process. This book covers these insights as well.

This book will be of value to both the student and the experienced practitioner. There are plenty of topics to dive into and practical tips to try out, and as Kortleve repeatedly emphasises, practice with patients will help you find an easier path through the diverse challenges faced in physiotherapy.

Professor Stephen Rollnick
Honorary Distinguished Professor,
School of Medicine, Cardiff University, United Kingdom

by Jeremy Lewis

Vincent Kortleve has trained as a physiotherapist and has studied psychology. He has also spent most of the 21st century working in primary care as a physiotherapist, as well as providing communication training for physiotherapists in the Netherlands and Belgium. He is both a clinician and an educator, and he has clearly used the expert skills he has mastered in both fields in a complementary fashion when crafting this book. His skills and knowledge will now be accessible to physiotherapists outside the Netherlands, helping to support and improve healthcare practice beyond the first publication of this work. We are indebted to Vincent for the time and energy he has devoted to writing *Communication Skills for Physiotherapists*, and for the information and guidance he has woven into every page of his book.

Via the book's 5 parts and 23 chapters, Vincent skilfully guides his target audience, clinical physiotherapists, through the complexity of communicating empathetically, respectfully, and effectively with people seeking care. On every page, Vincent has one clear focus: improving the way we listen to and converse with patients. He clearly recognises that the most important person in healthcare is the patient and that how we communicate at each stage of every meeting and interaction is crucial to developing a deep, broad, and meaningful therapeutic alliance. This book was originally published in Dutch, and we are fortunate that the publisher, Elsevier, is now releasing this valuable text in English. We are indebted to those who have translated this version into English.

Vincent correctly maintains that professional conversations may be difficult and need to be worked at to develop fully, as is necessary for every clinical skill. Practicing and refining the skills required to engage in meaningful professional conversations is the work of a lifetime; our communications abilities can always be improved. As such, this book will be invaluable for physiotherapists in training, those newly qualified, and those who have years (and years) of experience alike.

For this book to provide its intended benefit, it must not remain in the pristine condition in which it arrived in your hands. It demands that its pages should be well thumbed, filled with sticky notes, annotated by the reader, and discussed with colleagues and patients. The information within its pages should be reflected upon and compared with new research as it emerges.

Chapter 1, 'Before You Start', is the foundational chapter of the book and, as Vincent states, readers must resist the urge to skip or skim this section, as the book builds steadily from the information provided in the five concepts that are explained within.

As you dive into the book, you will become aware of the four roles that Vincent ascribes to the clinician when communicating: confidant, coach, communicative detective, and teacher. Each of these roles has its own specific characteristics.

In Chapter 3, Vincent describes the two different processes that occur during physiotherapy consultation: the diagnostic and therapeutic processes. He then identifies seven core tasks that are required for these processes to be most effective.

Within the book, Vincent provides suggestions and guidance on dealing with time pressures; how and when to use open and closed questions; how to build and maintain trust within the therapeutic relationship; the importance of non-verbal communication; the do's and don'ts of taking notes during the consultation; how to gather information and consent; using clinical language; engaging in patient education; and so much more. The book is a treasure trove filled with great advice and information. The consultation chapter clearly states, 'You never get a second chance to make a first impression', and then takes the reader through ways of making a positive first impression. The chapter on shared decision-making, goal-setting, and planning provides structure and guidance, as well as myriad suggestions to support clinical communication during these complicated and difficult processes.

Getting communication right during treatment is fraught with difficulty and ending a treatment session is not always straightforward. How do you deal with complications related to trust in the professional relationship? How do you keep the patient motivated? How can you use communication to improve self-efficacy and self-management? How do you communicate information about pain and how do you influence illness perceptions about pain with patients? If you have ever experienced difficulties with any of these issues or have ever been uncertain about how to best communicate any of these issues, you will be delighted with the suggestions for practice in this book.

Other strengths of the book include advice on how to communicate alternative information that may be quite different to the patient's perceptions, use metaphors in communication, and make comparisons in innovative ways—all important communication skills for any healthcare practitioner.

Depression occurs in 6% of the world's population and anxiety disorders in 8%. Chapter 16 presents strategies for communicating with people experiencing mental health disorders. Chapter 17 provides suggestions for communication between people from different cultures, as well as ideas for communicating when there are language barriers or challenges with a patient's health literacy skills. There is also a section on communicating with children of different ages and guidance on communicating with older members of society, as well as people suffering from dementia and those who may have intellectual disabilities. There are suggestions for effective ways of communicating with people who are deaf and those who are blind.

The book also includes suggestions for communicating risk, potential harms, and unwelcome news. It covers ways of discussing the relationship between the patient's lifestyle and their health concern, and offers suggestions to communicate and support lifestyle change.

The final section, Part V, focusses on scientific research and, in a similar fashion to the rest of the book, approaches the communication process in this area via the four roles outlined in the beginning: the clinician as a confidant, coach, communicative detective, and teacher.

In summary, *Communication Skills for Physiotherapists* is filled with detailed information, clear examples, and fantastic tips to improve every physiotherapist's skill when communicating with the most important person in healthcare, the patient. It is comprehensive and easy to read. There is valuable information on every page of this book, and everyone reading it will come away as a better communicator.

Jeremy Lewis PhD FCSP
Consultant Physiotherapist, National Health Service, United Kingdom
Professor of Musculoskeletal Research, University of Herefordshire, United Kingdom
Professor of Musculoskeletal Research, University of Limerick, Ireland
www.DrJeremyLewis.com

'This book had to be published'.

I wrote this in the Preface to the first Dutch edition of this book in the Netherlands, back in 2016. It took me more than three years to write that first Dutch edition; an important topic in a field like physiotherapy deserved a good treatment, and I wanted it to be a good read, not just another dry manual. Yet my intent was to write an approachable book that nevertheless did not describe the theme lightly, especially from a research and daily practice perspective. It was, and is, my mission to give professional communication the attention it deserves as a crucial competence in helping patients. Not for a moment did I think that an English version would ever appear, though I sometimes dreamed of it. I am so happy and proud that it is finally here in your hands!

Why did this book have to be published? For three reasons: First of all, to support active physiotherapists in their conversations with patients. Many of them are looking for (more) effective ways to approach and talk to their patients. I hope that with the help of the suggestions in this book, they will be able to take steps in this direction.

Second, I wrote this book for students who are training or specialising as physiotherapists. Physiotherapists in training, including those in undergraduate, graduate, and postgraduate programs, want to acquire or improve their professional knowledge and skills. This book can serve as a handbook for patient-clinician communication.

Last, but not least, it is all about the patients. Professional communication helps people to become and stay healthy, promote insight and understanding, decide together, motivate to change, and mobilise their resilience. With this book, I hope to contribute to those worthy goals.

Happy reading!

Vincent Kortleve

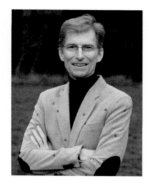

Vincent Kortleve is a physiotherapist who has also studied psychology. His great passion lies in human behaviour, particularly in influencing it effectively and respectfully through communication.

Vincent has spent almost his entire career working in education and in primary healthcare as a physiotherapist. Since 2006, he has worked as a trainer/teacher within his own company, Viaperspectief. He provides courses in the field of interviewing in the Netherlands and Belgium for small and large healthcare institutions, for various course providers, and for various physiotherapy master's programmes.

ACKNOWLEDGMENTS

To create this English edition, the first Dutch edition has been thoroughly updated. The people who helped me with the first Dutch edition, and whom I would like to thank, are Maarten Bijma, Max Lak, Maaike Kragting, Matijs van den Eijnden, Martin Moons (editing), Wilma de Hoog (text editing), and Heidi Kortleve (final editing).

Elsevier has performed the translation into English. It had to be an extremely accurate job, not least because many language nuances play a role in any conversation. I have often not made it easy for the team that did the translation. Thank you very much to everyone for your patience and commitment.

In recent years, many health professionals have shown a great deal of interest in conversations. Approaches such as 'shared decision-making' and 'motivational interviewing' are forms of conversation which have become mainstays in the curricula of (para)medical training and in continuing and furthering education. This tendency is also prevalent in physiotherapy; the important role that professional conversations play in physiotherapy is becoming increasingly clear.

In order to be able to describe conversations clearly and comprehensibly, so that a common theme emerges, different approaches and models from the literature on how to conduct conversations have been integrated with each other in this book. The most important models used are the roles described by Lang and van der Molen (Kortleve, 2006; G. Lang & van der Molen, 2014) and the core tasks worked out by Silverman (Silverman *et al.*, 2013). The 'four habits model' (Frankel & Stein, 1999) can also be recognised in the model described in this book.

To be most effective, physiotherapy care must be structured (Donaghy & Morss, 2000; Mann *et al.*, 2009; Plack & Greenberg, 2005)—that is, targeted, conscious, systematic, and process-based (Brouwer *et al.*, 1995). Of course, the same applies to physiotherapy conversations as a pathway to achieve adequate care. But doing so isn't simple. In order to systematically conduct your conversation with your patient, you must be aware of your own habits, weaknesses, and qualities. You have to be conscious of conducting the conversation in a structured manner, so that you can achieve the intended purpose of a part or of the whole conversation effectively and efficiently. You also need to be sufficiently flexible in your communication skills—human communication is erratic and complex.

This makes holding a professional, structured conversation a challenge. Yet this challenge should not take a back seat to our (justified) attention to clinical reasoning and 'technical' conduct in physiotherapy. In this sense, this is indeed a complex book! Physiotherapy conversations must take centre stage alongside other physiotherapy competencies of the primary process. Numerous scientific studies indicate that professional conversations deserve this position: improved self-management, stronger patient participation, better treatment results, improved therapy compliance, increased patient satisfaction, and more are our potential rewards. Here, we'll regularly refer to these studies; Part V of this book contains four chapters summarising purely scientific evidence in order to make it clear just how important conversation really is.

In an increasing number of countries, the description of skills for physiotherapists is based on the CanMEDS model (*Essential Competency Profile for Physiotherapists in Canada*, 2009; *Physiotherapy Competencies for Physiotherapy Practice in New Zealand*, 2009; 'Royal College of Physicians and Surgeons of Canada: CanMEDS', Zotero). This model emphasises the important role communication plays as a competency, and this book emphasises connecting with the CanMEDS model. I also pursued a link with the way in which Machteld Huber defined the concept of health (Huber *et al.*, 2011), as well as the biopsychosocial model of health (Engel, 1977).

In this book, physiotherapy conversations are developed within the primary process—that is, during the conversation that takes place between the physiotherapist and the patient in the consultation. Conversations with other health professionals in consultation situations, such as with inter- or intradisciplinary collaboration, are not described here.

This book is about *how*, as a physiotherapist, you communicate effectively with a patient and *why*. Sometimes this makes it necessary to look briefly at models which originate from health psychology, such as models related to illness perceptions or behavioural change. These models can help you, as a reader, to communicate professionally, and knowing about them can make this easier.

ACQUIRING COMMUNICATION SKILLS

The most important thing to remember for acquiring communication skills is that practice makes perfect! When observing skilled conversationalists, it often seems like this is an easy and natural thing—and therefore simple to learn. In reality, these people have often practised their skills for years in all kinds of situations, gaining ground and improving in conversational ability by learning the hard way. It's not something you can do just like that. Having a conversation can sometimes look so 'logical' and simple that it seems unnecessary to study it in depth in order to conduct a 'professional conversation'—let alone devote a whole book to it. This book assumes the opposite: conducting a professional conversation is critical and very tricky to carry out. Practice remains necessary, for everyone.

Systematic Approach

Wherever possible in this book, systems or step-by-step plans are presented. This was done in order to be able to work systematically and to meet the needs of many (future) physiotherapists, namely something to hold onto in practice. It is, of course, not obligatory to follow such a step-by-step plan or system. Sometimes the explanation in a paragraph will be enough for you to understand the meaning and implementation and you won't need the detailed plan. But sometimes an explanation is not enough: you know what it is trying to say, but it doesn't give you enough to act on. In such a case, it may be helpful to make use of the step-by-step plan provided. As you become more adept at an approach, you can abandon the step-by-step plan and choose your own pathway.

Online Environment

Additional material which supports/supplements parts of this book has been hosted on Evolve. Refer to the inside front cover page of this book for access information.

READING GUIDE

This book consists of five parts:
- **Part I** deals with a number of aspects of conducting a conversation which are useful to know before talking to patients. Think about your attitude to the patient during your conversation with them, or the 'roles' you often play implicitly while communicating with them.
- **Part II** discusses aspects which require ongoing consideration throughout the conversation. Think about the structure of the conversation, the relationship with your patient, and keeping them involved and engaged during the conversation.
- **Part III** describes the development of physiotherapy consultation from the first patient contact up to the conclusion of the course of therapy. It describes an ideal approach to the conversation with everything running smoothly and easily.
- **Part IV** deals with a variety of situations that may present issues in communicating with your patient. The usual approach as described in Part III may fall short; Part IV guides you on how to adapt or proceed.
- **Part V** is the last part and comprises a scientific account of the way in which communication is developed in this book. Regular reference is also made to scientific publications in Parts I to IV. However, in order to keep Parts I to IV easy to read, it has been written concisely, with a more extensive explanation of the research in Part V.

After long deliberation, for the sake of readability and as a result of a number of studies (Deber *et al.*, 2005; Kleinveld-Middelkoop & Peters, 2015), it was decided to use the word 'patient' in this book, instead of 'client'. 'Patient' seems to be the best way to express the patient's vulnerability in a physiotherapy consultation. Where the term 'patient' is used, it may also refer to the parents/carers or caregivers involved. Additionally, for ease of reference and inclusivity, 'they', 'their', and 'them' were used, both for the patient and for the physiotherapist.

PART I

Before You Start...

In this first part, the basic principles of physiotherapy conversations are examined. Chapter 1 describes the attitude with which you (subconsciously) approach your patient and which largely determines the effect of your communication. This attitude is the foundation for working with patients. Chapter 2 then discusses the four roles which you take on as a physiotherapist during your interaction with the patient. These roles are a common theme in this book because they create a specific framework regarding what, why, and how you communicate with your patient.

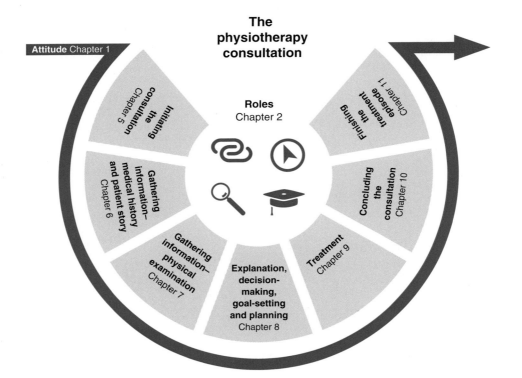

Attitude in Physiotherapy Conversations

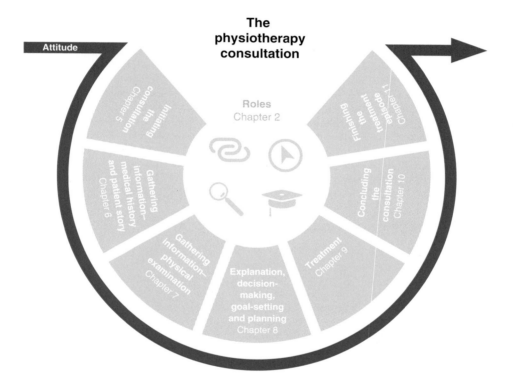

The physiotherapy consultation

Attitude

Initiating the consultation
Chapter 5

Gathering information–medical history and patient story
Chapter 6

Gathering information–physical examination
Chapter 7

Explanation, decision-making, goal-setting and planning
Chapter 8

Treatment
Chapter 9

Concluding the consultation
Chapter 10

Finishing the treatment episode
Chapter 11

Roles
Chapter 2

Communication between people is something special. The way in which you communicate with someone implicitly or explicitly shows them what you think about them or their behaviour. In other words, your communication always reveals your attitude. Attitude here is understood as a mix of your perceptions and your approach, or your stance in relation to the patient and the assistance you offer.

You may have an urge to quickly page through to the next chapter. Try to suppress this. All the techniques, step-by-step plans, and methods you will find in this book are based on 'attitude' as described in this chapter—it's essential foundational reading.

You will probably recognise the following scenario from your own life. Imagine you don't like someone. You don't appreciate the things they tell you in the same way you would have if you *did* like them—your attitude here determines how you take their remark. The same applies if you ask a question. Take, for example, the question, 'Why do you do that?' If your attitude when asking this question is suspicious, it is likely to come across in your intonation, and this question will sound different than when you ask it out of pure interest. Your posture, too, may change from being open with someone you like, to closed and distant with someone you don't. As you can see, your attitude comes through in your verbal and non-verbal communication alike.

In fact, your attitude often determines the final effect of your communication. Good communication skills without the right attitude are deceptive and therefore 'powerless' or ineffective. It's as if you're watching a movie with a good story, but played by bad actors—you will quickly lose interest. Your patient will almost certainly do the same. This book therefore starts with the attitude you have as a physiotherapist in communicating with your patient.

In order to circumscribe the tricky concept of 'attitude' in the physiotherapy context, this has been expanded in the next section to address a number of concepts of the provision of care and communication. These concepts take the form of statements. In the section that follows, you will read more about the skills needed to shape these concepts, known as attitude skills.

CONCEPTS OF CAREGIVING AND COMMUNICATION

In your work as a physiotherapist, you act on the basis of a number of views about health and illness, the patient, and interpersonal communication. You're not always aware of this.

In several countries, the professional competency profiles for physiotherapists give a description of caregiving, exercise, and health which is appropriate to the occupational profession of physiotherapy (*Essential Competency Profile for Physiotherapists in Canada*, 2009; *Physiotherapy Competencies for Physiotherapy Practice in New Zealand*, 2009; *Physiotherapy Practice Thresholds in Australia and Aotearoa New Zealand*, 2015; Owen & Hunter, 2015; Vries *et al.*, 2014). Central to this description is the biopsychosocial model. It goes without saying that this book does not diverge from this description.

Furthermore, you will find below five concepts which form the basis for physiotherapy communication as described in this book.

1. As a care worker, I focus on my partnership with the patient and act from the belief that the patient has the need:
   a) to understand their health problem and to look for logical links to explain it;
   b) to know what they can do to solve, reduce, or otherwise deal with their health problem.
2. As a care worker, I help the patient to make choices based on their own values and I hold the patient responsible for solving their health problem.
3. In the balance between vulnerability and resilience, I support the patient in fully addressing their personal competencies.
4. By investigating and strengthening the autonomous motivation of the patient, I enable the patient to change their behaviour in a sustainable way.
5. Professional physiotherapy communication is structured (targeted, systematic, process-based, and conscious) and based on scientific evidence ('evidence-based').

It's good to let these concepts sink in. It's quite a lot to digest! Read them again, one at a time, and imagine you're a patient. You have a sore knee or neck, or you have a chronic condition such as chronic obstructive pulmonary disease (COPD); you may have had an injury, so bear this in mind. Try now to think from the patient's perspective: Is this what you expect from a physiotherapist if you have an injury or a problem with movement?

A more detailed explanation of these five concepts, below, may help you better internalise these ideas from the perspective of both practitioner and patient.

Concept 1: A Partnership in Analysing and Resolving the Health Problem

Focusing on the patient is facilitated by a good relationship between the patient and the physiotherapist. The 'therapeutic alliance', i.e. cooperation between the patient and the physiotherapist, is of great importance for the result of the treatment (Duncan & Miller, 2000; Ferreira et al., 2013).

A person with a health problem will constantly look for a logical connection to explain their problem until they find one (Cameron & Leventhal, 2003). When the patient does not find a connection, they seek help from an expert. They expect the expert to contribute their knowledge and help them to discover and understand the connection without any self-interest (Deci & Vansteenkiste, 2004; Ryan & Deci, 2000). Attentive listening to the information the patient wants to convey is crucial. In fact, it is a case of two experts consulting with each other, on equal terms. The patient is an expert in their everyday life, beliefs, and feelings about their health and the things that are important to them. The professional, meanwhile, is an expert in their field, and is reasoning and acting from a biopsychosocial human perspective (Adler, 2009; Engel, 1977; Huber et al., 2011). Through professional patient-oriented communication, they bring their expertise and that of the patient together and search for a result that transcends the sum of the parts. Sensitivity to what exactly the patient says and means and how they express their thoughts and feelings is crucial. Your own behaviour and the way you express yourself verbally must also be carefully considered, as this is how you steer the conversation thoughtfully and systematically.

Concept 2: Making a Choice Based on One's Own Values and Taking Responsibility

By placing trust in the patient and their competencies, and working with them on an equal footing, with both of you being experts on the issue, you help the patient to use all their capabilities to solve their health problem. When dealing with specific aspects of the issue and as an expert in the area of functional movement, the physiotherapist takes more of a leading and guiding role. This is, after all, often the reason the patient is consulting the therapist—the patient's expertise is falling short. The therapist makes their expertise available to the patient, and the patient does with it what they want (Miller & Rollnick, 2012). Incidentally, this does not mean that the physiotherapist cannot and may not indicate their personal or professional boundaries.

In the end, the patient is the only one who knows what and how they want to solve their health problem, in a way that suits them and their values, or the things they find important (Rokeach, 1968; Ryan & Deci, 2000). This is clear from the decisions they make about treatment objectives and the treatment strategy (Scobbie et al., 2013). Such decision-making takes place in collaboration with the patient and in such a way that there is 'shared decision-making' (Edwards & Elwyn, 2009). Keeping this concept in mind while working with the patient, equal interaction becomes the primary feature of the collaboration.

Concept 3: Vulnerability and Resilience—Personal Competencies

Every patient with a health problem is off balance to some extent. This implies that they are vulnerable to a greater or lesser extent. Sometimes this vulnerability is immediately obvious; other times, you have the impression that there is no vulnerability at all. However, it is good to assume that every patient is vulnerable to some extent and to adjust your treatment accordingly (Brown, 2013).

At the same time, every patient is resilient, no matter how vulnerable. It is incredible how people can climb out of the depths of despair because of their resilience. You can appeal to this resilience in your interaction with your patient.

A calm and confident approach on your part helps the patient to show their vulnerability and also appeals to their resilience. Respect and acceptance are necessary. This also means that as a physiotherapist, you need to focus on the here and now. This is not always easy, as your phone, computer, and social media are all competing for your attention.

Concept 4: Autonomous Motivation

On a daily basis, physiotherapists are engaged with influencing the behaviour of their patients; for example, when giving advice, as well as assigning home exercises. Autonomous motivation, i.e. being motivated 'from the inside', is necessary to change behaviour in the long term or permanently (Ryan & Deci, 2000). A complicating aspect is that many people are ambivalent when it comes to changing their own behaviour (Prochaska *et al.*, 2013). Ambivalence in the patient can also arise if the physiotherapist provides information or instruction. The patient cannot or will not immediately believe the therapist, or may doubt whether the information applies to them. Ambivalence means that the situation often remains unchanged or the patient doesn't change their behaviour appropriately. Their opinion about certain matters remains the same, despite information or instruction from the physiotherapist.

It is one of the physiotherapist's tasks to help the patient to change (in behaviour or opinion). One way to do this is by helping the patient to explore their ambivalence. This allows the patient's autonomous motivation to emerge. Then, together with the physiotherapist, the patient can increase and strengthen that motivation. 'Change talk' plays an important role in this.

Concept 5: Structured Evidence-Based Communication

The actions of a professional such as a physiotherapist should be structured (Brouwer *et al.*, 1995; Mann *et al.*, 2009). Conducting a conversation is an essential part of physiotherapy treatment and should therefore also meet this requirement. Structured communication is systematic, process-based, conscious, and targeted.

The conversation with the patient is therefore conducted systematically, as the therapist knows what steps to take to achieve the set goal. They are aware of the effect their communication style can have and can adjust it if necessary (as it is process-based). If their communication proves to be ineffective, the therapist may deviate from their intended steps so that they still achieve their target in the conversation. The conversation is consciously controlled by the therapist and also consciously relinquished if necessary. The physiotherapist is able to reflect on the manner of their communication and its effectiveness.

In addition to conducting the conversation systematically, the physiotherapist should base it on scientific evidence. The chosen conversation techniques, the way in which the conversation is conducted, the approach to the patient and the underlying attitude—these are all based on scientific research evidence (Silverman *et al.*, 2013).

ATTITUDE SKILLS

The concepts discussed above influence your attitude and subsequent actions. Your attitude is formed around your skills, which is why it is called 'attitude skills' (Carkhuff, 1969).

The following attitude skills play a role in professional physiotherapy communication.

- **Empathy:** Empathy means that you view, hear and sense the world from the patient's frame of reference, as if you were the patient. You understand the patient's position without necessarily approving of their opinion and behaviour. You put into words what the patient wants to say. You empathise, listen carefully and reflect their thoughts and feelings.

- **Respect and acceptance:** Respect is shown by believing in the patient's capabilities and seeing the patient as a full collaborative partner in the process of care. You trust in the independence and self-reliance of the patient and believe in their ability to take responsibility without losing sight of their incapabilities. Acceptance means accepting the patient as they are, along with their qualities and weaknesses, and that you realise that everyone has attractive and less attractive sides to their personalities, just like you. Also, that they want to make their own choices and want to be enabled to do so. You listen patiently, make a shared decision and confirm each other's competencies.

- **Concreteness:** Concreteness means that you enable the patient to be specific about their feelings, thoughts and experiences. You help them articulate their feelings in such a way that they become understandable, to themselves as well as to you. You connect with the patient's way of thinking, enable them to gain knowledge and help them to process it. You speak plainly, ask (open) questions, do a recap, ponder the meaning and offer an explanation.

- **Genuineness:** Being genuine means that you stay true to yourself in the exchange, so that patients can also be themselves. You're authentic, sincere, open and assertive. This means that you are serious about what you say and do, that you show genuine interest, give real compliments and are truly involved with the patient. Genuineness also means bringing up appropriate personal experiences which can help the patient. Finally, being genuine means representing something: you know and manage your own limits, and those of your profession and of society.

Summary

- In communicating with the patient, the physiotherapist's attitude is decisive.
- The physiotherapist's attitude in the communication process comprises five concepts and four attitude skills.

However important, the physiotherapist's attitude should remain relatively abstract and requires concreteness. In any case, the next step is to give shape to four roles in the physiotherapy discussion. These roles are a common theme in this book and will be discussed in the next chapter.

The Four Roles in a Conversation

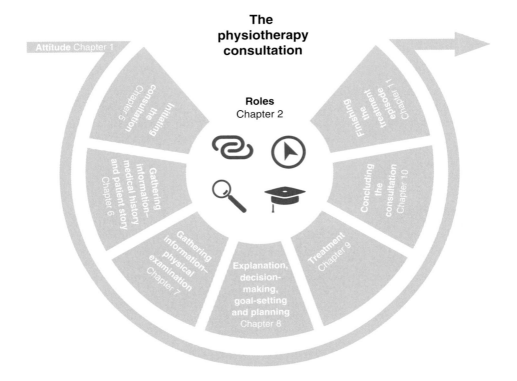

The physiotherapy consultation

Attitude Chapter 1

Initiating the consultation Chapter 5

Gathering information– medical history and patient story Chapter 6

Gathering information– physical examination Chapter 7

Explanation, decision-making, goal-setting and planning Chapter 8

Treatment Chapter 9

Concluding the consultation Chapter 10

Finishing the treatment episode Chapter 11

Roles
Chapter 2

In everyday life, everybody takes on different roles, often at the same time. An example of this is a man who trains a group of youths at a sports club. His overall role is that of a trainer. In addition, he sits on the technical committee (TC) responsible for classifying teams and selecting players. His role is therefore also as a TC member. In his role as a trainer, he has the youths do training exercises, while at the same time, in his role as a TC member, he observes which athletes have the qualities to play on the selection team.

As a physiotherapist, you also have different roles, including in a communicative sense. A description of these roles gives a clear picture of the attitude described in the previous chapter. It provides insight on what you do while conducting your conversation and on what you are to the patient. It also makes it possible to use your roles more purposefully and effectively. Such descriptions are also useful when you want to reflect on your own actions and when you want to have your conversation evaluated by others.

This book distinguishes four roles in communication (Kortleve, 2006; Lang & Van der Molen, 2014): confidant, coach, communicative detective, and teacher (Figure 2.1).

The role that you take on as a physiotherapist strongly depends on your patient's needs. The patient's needs are those things which the patient requires from the physiotherapist at a specific point in the conversation. Often, identifying these is more implicit than explicit. The physiotherapist will therefore have to be attentive to what the patient needs and/or seems to want to say. On that basis, you can choose their role and adapt it when necessary.

Each role has five characteristics:

- **The communication style of the physiotherapist:** This style describes the way of working and/or communication of the physiotherapist.
- **Content and/or process (Silverman *et al.*, 2013) skills:** Content skills relate to those skills which are expressed in words. Process skills are focused on the relationship and the way in which the patient and the physiotherapist work with each other. In short: the 'what' (content) and the 'how' (process) of the skills used.
- **The degree of directiveness:** The physiotherapist is directive if they steer the conversation substantially. The physiotherapist is non-directive if they don't steer, and instead leave it to the patient.

	CONFIDANT	COACH	COMMUNICATIVE DETECTIVE	TEACHER
Patient's Request	'Listen to me'	'Guide me'	'Help me to understand'	'Explain to me'
Communication Style	Following	Guiding	Offering	Explaining
Content and/or Process Skills	Process ⟵		⟶	Content
Directiveness	Non-Directive ⟵		⟶	Directive
Job-Specific Expertise	Absent ⟵		⟶	High
Attitude Skills	Empathy, Respect and Acceptance	Empathy, Respect And Acceptance, Concreteness	Respect and Acceptance, Concreteness, Genuineness	Concreteness and Genuineness

Figure 2.1 The four roles of the physiotherapist in the conversation.

- **The degree of job-specific expertise contributed by the physiotherapist:** This expertise concerns specific knowledge and insight from the professional physiotherapy domain.
- **The attitude skills:** Although all the attitude skills appear in all four roles, these skills stand out in particular.

The four roles are explained in more detail in the following paragraphs.

THE PHYSIOTHERAPIST AS CONFIDANT

In order to provide adequate care, the physiotherapist acts as a confidant (Ferreira *et al.*, 2013; Mauksch *et al.*, 2008; Pinto *et al.*, 2012). In this way, the trust-based relationship between the physiotherapist and the patient becomes central, and the therapist is non-directive: the patient determines the conversation while the therapist creates structure and rest. They accept the patient as a human being, respecting their qualities and weaknesses. They try to understand the patient and their environment and to imagine themselves in their position. Job-specific knowledge and skills are not required here; the patient mainly requires a listening ear from someone they can trust. In fact, a neighbour or friend could also take on this role. The role of confidant makes it possible for the physiotherapist to effectively assume their other roles.

The physiotherapist acts in this role on the basis of the attitude skills of empathy, respect, and acceptance; they create warmth, safety, and trust, and listen in order to understand.

THE PHYSIOTHERAPIST AS COACH

In the role of coach, the physiotherapist appeals to the self-regulating capacity (and self-management) of the patient. They help the patient to change their behaviour, while eliciting and strengthening an autonomous motivation. In order to achieve a behavioural change (e.g. regular exercises), the patient is guided by the physiotherapist in such a way that they retain control. The physiotherapist explores with the patient their ambivalence towards changing and helps to reduce it to benefit the intended change. They enable the patient to investigate and strengthen their own motivation by selectively eliciting and strengthening change talk without convincing the patient or imposing choices (Miller & Rollnick, 2012). When solving problems, they support and stimulate the patient in such a way that they fully address and use their own capabilities. They allow the patient to find themselves, don't influence the discovery directly, and guide the patient towards what they are looking for. Both content and process skills play a role in communication. In this, the physiotherapist makes limited use of their job-specific expertise.

In this role, the physiotherapist acts on the basis of the attitude skills of empathy, respect and acceptance, and concreteness.

THE PHYSIOTHERAPIST AS COMMUNICATIVE DETECTIVE

As an expert in the field of health problems in human movement, the physiotherapist constantly analyses the things the patient says and does. The clinical reasoning process is central to this. In clinical reasoning, the physiotherapist operates as a detective (Ahlsen *et al.*, 2018). Clinical reasoning, however, is not a solitary activity. The patient also tries to analyse their health problem and is thus familiar with a (clinical) reasoning process (Leventhal *et al.*, 2003). During the physiotherapy consultation, the patient asks, explicitly or implicitly, for the physiotherapist's help with their own analysis and reasoning process so that they can start to understand their health problem. Where possible, the physiotherapist will share their analysis with the patient on the basis of their expertise, and present what they are thinking about in order to further assist the patient's analysis process. The physiotherapist now takes on the role of communicative detective.

For the physiotherapist, clinical reasoning is a search for the type and extent of the patient's health problem and its solution. They constantly interact with the patient to obtain relevant information to guide their clinical reasoning. In this way, they try to get a clear picture of the patient's (sometimes dysfunctional) way of thinking, feeling, and acting with regard to their health problem, and of the possible anatomical, medical, psychological, psychophysiological, and sociological aspects of their health problem. They conduct the conversation in such a way that all relevant themes are addressed in sufficient depth, while at the same time giving the patient room to contribute their own thoughts, reasoning, and interpretations. The physiotherapist shares their reasoning with the patient, involving them in their analyses, explaining these, and providing the patient with interim and final conclusions. They give the patient the opportunity to react to their findings and influence these, without allowing the conversation to become less effective. Ultimately, they come to a shared decision with the patient about treatment goals and strategies.

Again, the conversation is a dialogue: both interlocutors have their own and specific input, work closely together, and complement each other. This is in contrast to an interview in which the patient is subjected to an 'interrogation' and the therapist 'demands' all the information. The conversation and the skills of the communicative detective are focused more on the content than on the process.

In this role, the physiotherapist acts on the basis of the attitude skills of respect and acceptance, concreteness, and genuineness.

■ Using the Roles

Among other things, the roles in this chapter have a didactic value. As an undergraduate physiotherapist or novice, you are trying to find your footing in daily practice, as well as in your conversations. The four roles give you a foundation to hang onto, without acting as a straitjacket.

Of course, you hardly ever use one role in isolation; often, you will combine roles when talking to patients. However, it may be good to concentrate on one role at a time at the beginning of your training. As you gain more experience, you can then alternate and/or combine roles.

The roles can also be used as a tool for evaluation retrospectively. You can then ask yourself which role was needed at a specific point in the conversation, which role you decided to adopt, and whether you were successful or not.

THE PHYSIOTHERAPIST AS TEACHER

The physiotherapist often explains things to the patient, such as knowledge and insight concerning the health problem, an exercise, a technique they are going to perform, and so on. In this, the role of teacher is recognisable (Cooper et al., 2009; Engers et al., 2008; King et al., 2018; Mosley & Butler, 2017).

In this role, the physiotherapist works with a certain directiveness. This is expressed, among other things, by the firmness with which the teacher provides the information. If the information is well substantiated from literature and/or research in the job-specific context, it can be presented more firmly. If the substantiation is inadequate or absent, the physiotherapist should present the information less firmly. In the role of teacher, the directiveness can also depend on the therapeutic objective(s). Think, for example, of a situation in which meticulous instruction is appropriate to the therapeutic objective(s). The physiotherapist always fulfils this role while respecting the patient's autonomy, and in cooperation with the patient.

In this role, the physiotherapist mainly acts on the basis of the attitude skills of concreteness and genuineness.

Summary

In this second chapter, four roles are elaborated:

- The physiotherapist as a confidant listens by bringing clarity and calmness to the connection, showing attention and understanding for the patient's experiences and encouraging the patient to speak freely.
- As coach, the physiotherapist acts as a guide to the patient in the conversation so that the patient makes full use of their own personal capabilities and autonomous motivation to change their behaviour to achieve the desired effect.
- In interaction with the patient, the physiotherapist as communicative detective tries to obtain a clear picture of all aspects of the health problem in order to bring about a professional, clinical reasoning process. To this end, the physiotherapist asks questions while giving the reason for and the intention of those questions, informing the patient about their (interim) conclusions and reflecting on them in consultation with the patient. They finally make a shared decision.
- The physiotherapist as a teacher gives the patient a better perspective of their health problem, while respecting their autonomy. They also inform and educate the patient about their health problem and its solution, and they instruct the patient in the execution of an agreed treatment goal.

PART II

During the Conversation

The foundation for professional communication—your attitude as a physiotherapist—has now been laid. In order to arrive at concrete action within the physiotherapy consultation, Chapter 3 discusses the seven core tasks which indicate what the physiotherapist has to do during the diagnostic and therapeutic process. Within these core tasks, the physiotherapist fulfils the roles of confidant, coach, communicative detective, and teacher.

Further along in Chapter 3, you will read about 'thought structures'. This helps you structure the content of the conversation; in other words, it helps you determine what the conversation is about.

When you start a conversation with your patient, you have to pay attention to certain elements throughout the whole conversation, from beginning to end. You need to think about building and maintaining the relationship with your patient and providing structure. These aspects, which are independent of the core task, are discussed in Chapter 4.

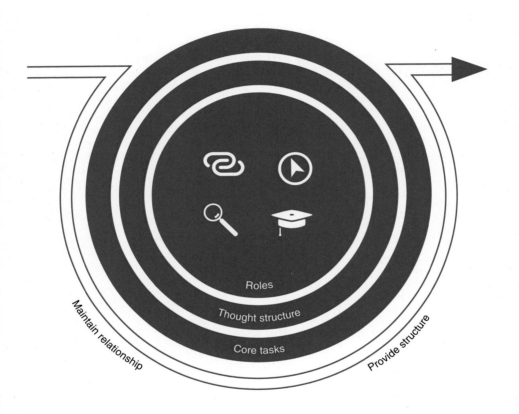

CHAPTER 3

The Seven Core Tasks in the Conversation

CORE TASKS

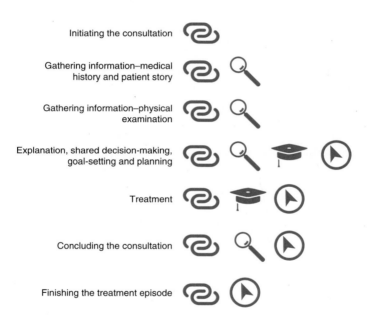

Initiating the consultation

Gathering information–medical history and patient story

Gathering information–physical examination

Explanation, shared decision-making, goal-setting and planning

Treatment

Concluding the consultation

Finishing the treatment episode

During each physiotherapy consultation, the physiotherapist has seven core tasks. These form the basis of every professional consultation and guide them as they are happening (Silverman, 2014). As a physiotherapist, you use a content-based discussion format during the execution of these core tasks, referred to as a 'thought structure' in this book. A thought structure consists of a list of topics that you want to include in the conversation and about which you want to find out more from the patient. A thought structure helps you to make sure you don't forget topics during a conversation.

SEVEN CORE TASKS

The physiotherapy consultation has two different processes: the diagnostic process and the therapeutic process (Vries *et al.*, 2014). During the diagnostic process, the patient's health problem is analysed and a shared decision is made about the treatment to pursue. The therapeutic process involves carrying out and planning the treatment, and monitoring the treatment results.

According to Silverman (Silverman *et al.*, 2013), seven core tasks can be distinguished in the conversation with the patient within the diagnostic and therapeutic process:
1. Initiating the consultation
2. Gathering information—medical history and patient story
3. Gathering information—physical examination
4. Explanation, shared decision-making, goal-setting and planning
5. Treatment (incl. explanation, instruction, and education)
6. Concluding the consultation
7. Finishing the treatment episode

The aim of a consultation will determine which of the seven core tasks will be carried out. Core tasks 1 to 6 will usually be completed during an initial consultation, in which the diagnostic process is central. Depending on the results of the physiotherapy analysis and the decision-making process with the patient, the fifth core task is sometimes dropped. If treatment proceeds, follow-up consultations will mainly consist of core tasks 1, 4, 5, and 6, and to a much lesser extent, core tasks 2 and 3. Core task 7 is only relevant if physiotherapy treatment has taken place and the treatment programme is completed as a whole.

The core tasks only give a rough breakdown of your conversational tasks as a physiotherapist. Among other things, this classification has a didactic purpose and helps to divide the consultation into a few coherent chunks. How exactly you can fulfil these core tasks as a physiotherapist is laid out in detail in Chapters 4 to 11.

THE FUNCTION OF THE FOUR ROLES IN THE CORE TASKS

The roles discussed in Chapter 2 turn up once again in the different core tasks and give substance to the physiotherapy communication. Table 3.1 gives an overview of the relationship between the core tasks, the roles, and the possible thought structure (see the next section).

THE THOUGHT STRUCTURE IN THE CORE TASKS

During the consultation, the physiotherapist uses a thought structure within some core tasks; for example, in core task 2 (gathering information – medical and patient history). Such a thought structure consists of an overview of the aspects you want to gather information about during the consultation. In other words: a thought structure helps you with the question, 'What is the conversation about?' An example of a widely used thought structure is the International Classification of Functioning, Disability, and Health (ICF).

TABLE 3.1 ■ **The Connection Between the Core Tasks, the Roles and the Thought Structure**

Core Task	Role in the Conversation	Thought Structure
Initiating the consultation	Confidant	
Gathering information – medical & patient history	Confidant, Communicative detective	Screening
Gathering information – medical history & patient story	Confidant, Communicative detective	Medical & patient history
Gathering information – physical examination	Confidant, Communicative detective	
Explanation & shared decision-making	Confidant, Communicative detective	
Goal-setting & planning	Confidant, Communicative detective	
Treatment (incl. explanation, instruction and education) Concluding the consultation	Confidant, Coach, Teacher, Communicative detective	. Treatment
Concluding the treatment episode	Confidant, Coach, Communicative detective	

Bear in mind that a thought structure should not unnecessarily dominate and prescribe communication; on the contrary—deviating is the rule rather than the exception. The thought structure is mainly a reminder, not a list for you to work through point by point in your conversation. Moreover, the thought structure you use must fit in with the concepts described in Chapter 1 and the professional competence profile for physiotherapy. In this way, the thought structure must support the collection and analysis of biomedical and psychosocial elements of the health problem.

In this book, three thought structures are used: one for during the screening, one while taking the history, and one for during the follow-up or treatment consultation. Other thought structures, such as the ICF and the SCEBS (somatic, cognitive, emotional, behavioural, and social), can be found on Evolve. If you'd rather use those, please go ahead.

Thought Structure for Screening

If the patient has not been referred by a general practitioner but consults the physiotherapist directly, it is necessary to carry out a screening. During the screening, the physiotherapist determines whether there is a possible indication for physiotherapy (Heerkens *et al.*, 2012). In the screening process, the physiotherapist has to take on core tasks 1 to 4. Itemising the following in a thought structure would be helpful (with the core task of the physiotherapist in brackets):

- Explore the contact reason and/or request for help (core task 2).
- Screen the case as serious/not serious (core tasks 2 and 3):
    - assess for signs and symptoms;
    - assess for red flags.
- Provide information about the indication for further physiotherapy diagnostics, contact with a general practitioner, or a wait-and-see policy (core task 4).
- Shared decision-making with the patient (core task 4).

Thought Structure for Medical and Patient History

If it has been established that physiotherapy is (possibly) indicated, a further diagnostic process takes place (from core task 2). A clear and effective thought structure for the interview (core task 2) is the following (Staal *et al.*, 2013):

- Review the patient's request for help and their health problem:
  - request for help, changes in daily functioning, details of what the patient's request for help is based on (including in terms of disorders, limitations in activities, and partici-pation problems);
  - type and severity of the complaint;
  - symptoms, phenomena, signs, provocation, and/or reduction;
  - patient's view regarding type and severity (illness perceptions).
- Screen for 'red flags'
- Take stock of the patient's current health status:
  - current level of functioning (activities and participation);
  - impediments to recovery:
    - 'yellow flags';
    - patient's way of dealing with the problem—(a) patient's view on their health status (illness perceptions); (b) is the patient coping adequately with their pain and/or reduced functioning? (c) does the patient have a sense of control over their health problem? (d) what significance does the patient attach to their health problem?
    - general load and load capacity, and regional load and load capacity;
    - co-morbidity;
    - work-related factors.
- Determine the onset of the health problem, and the cause or causal factors:
  - time bar;
  - cause of the health problem:
    - traumatic: trauma analysis;
    - non-traumatic: relevant changes in load or load capacity (general, regional, and/or local);
  - function *before* the onset of the health problem (level of activity, degree of participation, load and load capacity);
  - patient's view on cause (illness perceptions);
  - psychosocial factors: stress, social, lifestyle, or behavioural factors.
- Review the medical and patient history:
  - the course of the health problem (normal or abnormal), influencing factors and the level of functioning;
  - (local, regional and general) load and (local, regional, and general) load capacity, both at the level of functions and at the level of activities and participation;
  - previous diagnostics and treatment and their results;
  - patient's view of the factors influencing the course of the health problem (illness perceptions);
  - psychosocial factors: stress, social, lifestyle, or behavioural factors.
- Review any other information:
  - health status (disorders, diseases);
  - current treatment, use of medication and aids, advice and aids;
  - contraindications for therapeutic intervention;
  - social aspects relating to work, housing, and family situation.

Thought Structure for 'Treatment'

The most common conversation, but the least conspicuous, takes place during the consultations dedicated to the treatment of the patient. The physiotherapist evaluates the result of the treatment(s) up to that point with the patient: is there progression, is progress as expected, are there setbacks, and so on. Together with the patient, they then determine the continuation of the treatment and proceed with that plan.

Here, too, a thought structure is useful. And again, this thought structure is also used flexibly: it is up to you which parts need to be included in the conversation and in what order. For example, exploring the course of the health problem and/or deviations from expectations will probably be discussed less thoroughly (or not at all) if it appears that recovery is taking place as expected.

The thought structure is as follows:

- Review the patient's current health status:
  - severity and type of complaints, current level of functioning (disorders, activities, and participation) in relation to sub-targets and main goal;
  - the way in which the health problem is being dealt with:
    - Is the patient coping adequately with their reduced functioning and/or pain?
    - Does the patient have a sense of control over their health problem?
    - What significance does the patient attach to their complaints?
- Review the course of the health problem:
  - in conjunction with the level of functioning;
  - in relation to (local and general) load and (local and general) load capacity, both at the level of function and at the level of activities and participation.
- In the case of deviation from expectations:
  - What is causing and/or explains the reduction in or lack of progression?
  - Are there any possible red flags?
  - Are there any possible yellow flags?

THE ELECTRONIC PATIENT RECORD

In recent years, for many physiotherapists, the physiotherapy conversation has been dominated by filling in the electronic patient record (EPR). The agenda or structure of the conversation during the diagnostic process is then determined by the design of the EPR software (i.e. the check boxes on the computer screen). This often leads to unwanted and frequent interruption in connecting with the patient because the physiotherapist is occupied with searching on their screen or busy typing (Margalit *et al.*, 2006; Silverman & Kinnersley, 2010). In addition, there are other disadvantages to using the EPR in such a way during a conversation.

- The physiotherapist follows the structure of the EPR instead of the patient's story. This disrupts the patient's story to such an extent that it may eventually lead to certain issues not being addressed: Think mainly of personal and relevant psychosocial information. The roles of confidant, coach, and communicative detective are muddled or lost.
- Care workers who use a computer while taking the history are missing relevant verbal and non-verbal information because of trying to do two things at once (Shachak *et al.*, 2009).
- The patient may not feel they are being taken seriously because the physiotherapist is more concerned with looking at their screen than with them (Silverman & Kinnersley, 2010).

In short, the electronic patient record is not a suitable structure to form part of the conversation and quickly disrupts communication.

Summary

During the conversation with the patient, the physiotherapist follows seven core tasks. These core tasks are a didactic tool to discuss and teach physiotherapy conversations in a structured way. In order to cover all the necessary topics, a thought structure is helpful as a reminder for the physiotherapist during the conversation. The EPR is unsuitable as a structure for conversation.

CHAPTER 4

Conversation Aspects Independent of the Core Task

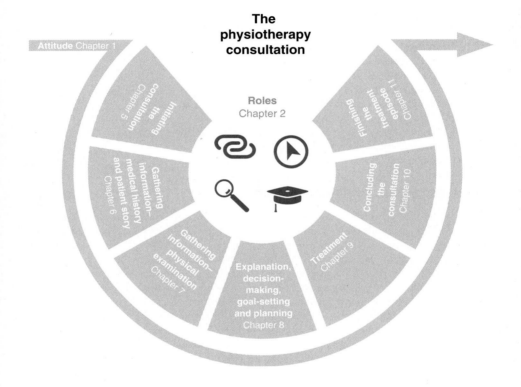

The conversation with the patient is about to begin. The physiotherapy conversation has a number of aspects which require your attention throughout the conversation and are therefore independent of the core task. These are an important task of the confidant. This involves 'providing structure', 'building and maintaining the relationship', (Silverman et al., 2013) and 'involving and keeping the patient involved'. By paying attention to these aspects, you are putting into action some of the principles discussed in Chapter 1.

PROVIDING STRUCTURE

By offering structure during the consultation (Cole & Bird, 2013; Pretorius *et al.*, 2010), the physiotherapist achieves the following objectives:
- all subjects are addressed and given the attention they deserve, both biomedically and psychosocially;
- the consultation is targeted, effective, and efficient;
- the patient gets clarity and uncertainty is avoided;
- the collaboration takes shape because patient and therapist know at every stage of the conversation what the goal is.

In the role of confidant, you create structure and safeguard it. You do this, for example, by summarising, explaining why you want to discuss a certain subject, and making step-by-step plans.

Of course, creating too rigid a structure during the consultation is not desirable. You might hold the patient back so they can't tell their own story. Relevant biomedical and especially psychosocial elements are often left out of the conversation. On the other hand, it is inadvisable to offer too little structure. This has partly the same result: an inadequate analysis of the health problem. Too little structure can also lead to time pressures if the conversation goes on without a clear focus.

Put Into Action: Providing Adequate Structure

As a confidant, you offer as much structure as is necessary. This requires sensitivity from the physiotherapist for what the patient wants to say and its relevance for the analysis. This is quite a challenge, especially with talkative patients. If you are a new physiotherapist, it is quite possible that you will hold on a bit more to the structure of the conversation, the systems, and the step-by-step plans provided in this book. As your experience increases, you almost certainly become more flexible and can consciously and purposefully deviate from it.

You offer structure (Silverman *et al.*, 2013) by doing the following:
- Choosing a logical structure for the conversation (such as using a thought structure, applying step-by-step plans, and using systems and models) and helping the patient to see when this is needed.
- Providing summaries (repeating concisely or comprehensively what the patient has said, both during and at the end of the conversation) and paraphrasing/reaffirming (briefly describing in your own words what the patient has said).
- Marking transitions in the conversation (by briefly indicating the next phase of the consultation, e.g. conducting a physical examination).
- Choosing a good time to link up with a patient's comment (e.g. by going deeper into psychosocial aspects of the health problem if the patient brings it up).
- Stating that you are deviating from the intended steps and why you are doing this.
- Metacommunicating by discussing how the conversation itself is going (e.g. if the communication is not optimal, you discuss this with the patient).
- Using explanatory illustrations or (anatomical) models, diagrams, and drawings (e.g. on a whiteboard or flip-over board).
- Thinking out loud (making the patient understand that it is good to pause with a specific theme and to look at it more closely).

Time Pressure

Sometimes it may be necessary to guide the structure of the conversation more firmly—for example, because the health problem is of a complex nature with a wide range of biomedical and psychosocial factors, or because you are running out of time and you know that the next patient is already waiting for you. In the latter case, you want to let the current patient know that you need to end the consultation without letting them feel that the things they have to say are unimportant. You could, for example, say: 'I notice there are still some issues you'd like to discuss with me. Unfortunately, we can't do that today because we're running out of time. I hope you understand that we will have to deal with these issues in our next consultation'.

Open and Closed Questions

The structure you offer also depends on the type of questions you ask. Many physiotherapists try to bring structure to the conversation by mainly asking closed questions. In this way, they take more of a 'leadership role' in the conversation, thereby giving it the semblance of structure. This has a few major disadvantages: namely, that you (strongly) restrict the patient's story and that the psychosocial and personal aspects of a health problem, in particular, are not given enough attention. It is better to ask open questions and to appropriately use directive questions. This makes it possible, even in the case of talkative patients, to give the conversation sufficient structure and at the same time give the patient sufficient opportunity to tell their own story.

An example of structuring by asking closed questions is: 'Is it painful when you bend your knee? What if you sit down? And stand up?' This type of structuring restricts the patient in telling their story and, in any case, the answer probably gives you only very limited information. Moreover, you often have to ask a lot of questions before you learn what you want to know. An alternative is an open question which is aimed at proceeding in a certain direction. For example: 'If we focus a little more on the times that you experience pain, when is that?' Or: 'Which activities cause you pain? (…) And which even more?'

■ Directive Questioning

By purposefully formulating your open questions, you can influence the direction of the conversation. This is directive questioning. An open question which is not very directive is, for example: 'What else can you tell me about your shoulder?' An open question which is very directive is: 'When do you think you are overloading your shoulder?' For the first question, the patient can determine the direction of their answer entirely by themselves: what they are going to tell you is up to them. For the second question, you are already leading the patient much more in a certain direction (i.e. the strain on their shoulder and how they think about it), but by still using an open question, you don't partly pre-empt the answer (as is often the case with a closed question).

Purposeful use of directive questioning leads to a more efficient and effective conversation. Use fewer directive questions if you want the patient to determine the direction (and you may be curious to know which direction the patient chooses). Use more if you want to learn more about a specific aspect.

In Consultation

Fewer directive questions	Is there anything else that's bothering you?
	Well, I don't believe there is. In my opinion, I think I've mentioned everything.
Providing structure	Mmm, just a few more short questions.
Strong directive question	To what extent do you experience tingling sensations in your forearm or hand?
	No, never had that.

In Consultation—cont'd

Moderate use of directive questions	What is the feeling like in your hand? *Um, just normal.*
Providing structure: mark transitions	All right. Now, I'd like to talk to you about the cause of your health problem. What can you tell me about that? *Well, I'm not sure, but I have an idea. I think…*

BUILDING AND MAINTAINING THE RELATIONSHIP

Building and maintaining the relationship with the patient is a crucial aspect of your role as a confidant. This role is a prerequisite for fulfilling the roles of coach, communicative detective, and teacher and you must therefore apply it to all consultations during all core tasks.

You and the patient work together during the first consultation and the follow-up consultations. There must be mutual trust and partnership. This is necessary because you want the patient to feel free to share with you as many aspects of their health problem as possible (including those which are personal) so that you can make an optimal analysis of their health problem. The collaboration also makes shared decision-making possible and plays a role in the patient following up on advice and therapy compliance.

Among other things, research into the relationship of trust between the physiotherapist or care worker and the patient shows that:

- patients follow up on advice sooner in a good relationship of trust (Derksen *et al.*, 2013; Van Dulmen, 2012);
- the 'therapeutic alliance'—the human connection between physiotherapist and patient— also determines the treatment effect (Ferreira *et al.*, 2013; Pinto *et al.*, 2012);
- the patient's satisfaction with the consultation is strongly related to a pleasant and empathic connection with the healthcare provider (Hall *et al.*, 1981, 1988; Pretorius *et al.*, 2010);
- therapists are more satisfied with their work and value their assistance more if they have a good relationship with the patient (Pretorius *et al.*, 2010; Silverman *et al.*, 2013), which in turn benefits the commitment and compassion of the therapist in the assistance process.

Day-to-day practice is tricky in this respect. For some care workers, the quality of the personal contact takes a back seat and the biomedical aspects of the health problem dominate the consultation, making the contact terse and business-like.

Put Into Action: Building and Maintaining the Relationship

Building and maintaining the relationship with the patient strongly depends on the physiotherapist's types of non-verbal and verbal behaviour. For example, literature shows that people like each other better if they 'mirror' each other (Dijksterhuis, 2011; Hinz, 2000; Strack & Förster, 2011). Mirroring refers to the adoption of a patient's non-verbal cues, such as their posture. In a verbal sense, this can also be done by, for example, using (almost) the same words as the patient. In addition, eye contact and an open attitude are very important for creating and maintaining a good relationship with the patient (Harrigan *et al.*, 1985; Pretorius *et al.*, 2010; Staveren, 2010).

Non-Verbal Communication

The most important types of non-verbal behaviour that help build and maintain a relationship of trust with your patient are:

- regular eye contact;
- an open posture;

- appropriate humming and nodding;
- smiling once in a while.

Another important aspect in the relationship is 'modelling', a concept that has been described extensively in the literature on neurolinguistic programming (NLP) (Dilts & Grinder, 1980). NLP often uses the term 'rapport' for this purpose. When you tune in to your patient, you try to communicate on the same wavelength. By adopting aspects of the patient's behaviour, you meet the human need to see something of yourself mirrored in the other person with whom you are in contact. If that need is met, people often experience the contact as satisfying and enjoyable; you and the patient understand each other and the conversation goes smoothly. Modelling—that is, *seemingly* imitating or mirroring the other person's behaviour—is something that people are already inclined to do of their own accord, albeit usually subconsciously. There are several types of non-verbal behaviour you can model (Dilts & Grinder, 1980; Hinz, 2000), namely:

- **body language:** mirroring part of the patient's body position or body movements;
- **mimicry (facial expressions):** for example, using your eyes to help express yourself when the patient does so too, or smiling when the patient also smiles;
- **voice and speech (speed, volume, pitch, intonation):** for example, adjusting your voice pitch, speaking speed, or accent towards that of the patient.

Modelling does not mean that you are trying to pretend to be the patient or that you identify with them. Rather, you are simply being yourself and engaging in non-verbal behaviour which benefits the relationship with your patient. Consciously participating in this may feel artificial, especially in the beginning. Modelling, however, is a powerful tool in the role of confidant.

■ 'Other' Sources of Trust

In building a relationship of trust with your patient, it can be good to also look at other aspects of communication. Think about the clothes you wear and the impression you make wearing that clothing. This, of course, depends on the context of your work and also on the customs and habits (culture) of the country and/or region in which you work. A general rule of thumb here is to appear clean and well-dressed, in a way that is acceptable to all patients (from young to old). Under no circumstances do you want your clothing to create 'distance' between you and the patient. That can be quite a challenge in some cases. Pay attention to the fact that your clothing always communicates something about you (Rufa'i et al., 2015; Mercer et al., 2008).

In addition, the layout of the room where you carry out your consultations is also important. Make sure, as far as you can, to create a warm, calm, and friendly atmosphere. Try to arrange your space in such a way that holding conversations with people, in addition to doing exercises, is as easy as possible. If you have photos or pictures on the wall, make sure that they convey a positive message about the human body and emphasise the trainability and resilience of the human being. Keep in mind that anatomical models and plates often focus on what's wrong; that might not be the image you want to portray to your patient.

Verbal Communication

Verbal behaviour is also important for the relationship with the patient. Central to this is recognising the patient's feelings and thoughts. By primarily *acknowledging* these and not directly refuting or wanting to change them (as can be indicated implicitly by reassuring someone), the patient feels that they are allowed the feelings and thoughts they have, as well as feeling that they themselves are allowed to be there. This creates a powerful supportive impulse for the relationship of trust. You can acknowledge the thoughts and feelings of the patient by:

- being genuinely curious about their thoughts or feelings by leaving time for them and by asking the patient about them;

- repeating, summarising, or reflecting the patient's thoughts or feelings;
- helping the patient to empathically express their thoughts or feelings (or the consequences thereof).

In all of this, suppress the tendency to say 'Yes, but…' or to immediately start looking for solutions.

Beyond this, verbal modelling is powerful. Much like behavioural modelling, this involves adopting aspects of the patient's speech and using images and metaphors also used by the patient and/or which fit in with their (apparent) perception of the world.

INVOLVING AND KEEPING THE PATIENT INVOLVED

Patient participation is becoming increasingly central in physiotherapy care. Patient participation is about the patient taking part in the process of care, not as a passive object but as a full partner. Patient participation goes hand in hand with strengthening self-management. Good patient self-management (especially in a chronic illness) results in a healthier patient who is less dependent on care providers and who (in some cases) incurs fewer costs in care. Patient participation also relates to autonomy. Autonomy is a core value for every human being. In the 'self-determination theory', it forms an important pillar (Ryan & Deci, 2000). Increasingly, autonomy is also a core value in all kinds of legislation in which the rights and duties of patients are defined.

An involved patient takes responsibility for their problem. This is crucial in physiotherapy care because people do not *undergo* a one-off intervention, often instead playing an active role in the recovery for a longer period of time.

Incidentally, many care workers think that the patient is unable to participate in numerous things and therefore often take control themselves, with the result that patient participation is nil. According to some care workers, patient participation is too difficult or too complicated. In this view, patients aren't able to help decide about certain matters and involving them would unnecessarily increase the costs of care. In reality, the opposite is true. Patients often make sensible choices and tend to solve many things themselves, as long as it is clear to them what is going on and what a suitable solution may be, or what the possibilities are (Oshima Lee & Emanuel, 2013; Stacey *et al.*, 2011). A prerequisite for good patient participation is that you have confidence in the patient's skills, listen carefully, and provide the patient with good, personalised information.

Keeping the patient involved during consultations is expressed in the role of the 'confidant' and affects all other roles.

Put Into Action: Involving and Keeping the Patient Involved

In order to involve and keep the patient involved during the consultation, the following five focal points are important:

1. Involve your patient from the start of the conversation;
2. Listen, in order to understand;
3. Keep the 'information gap' as narrow as possible;
4. Attune to the patient's use of language;
5. Ask personal questions.

The first focal point, to involve the patient from the start of the conversation, seems obvious but is not self-evident in practice. Involving the patient from the start avoids putting them in a passive and dependent role. You more or less 'define' your role and that of the patient in the first few minutes of the consultation, setting the tone for the next consultation and even those thereafter.

The second point also sounds logical and simple: listen. But there is a key addition: *in order to understand*. And that might make this harder than it looks. A common pitfall when listening is that you do so from your own frame of reference or 'filter'. So you mainly hear what you want to hear—and maybe not always what the patient wants to say or what they mean. Listening to the other person is therefore a way of connecting with what the other person means to say. This essential skill is further discussed in Chapter 6.

The third point boils down to giving information at the right time, thereby being communicative. During the initial interview, you analyse the patient's health problem. Many physiotherapists only share their insights after taking the history and at the end of the physical examination. However, by regularly sharing your analysis and (interim) conclusions with your patient while interviewing the patient and conducting the examination (i.e. telling the patient what you are thinking about and what connections you see), the patient becomes more involved. You will also notice that the patient tends to share your thoughts and 'co-analyse' more. And that's exactly what you want to achieve. Of course, you will be selective in the information you give, and it is important to formulate your analysis or conclusion and adapt its forcefulness to that point in time. But if you are sufficiently communicative, the patient will enhance the analysis process by being more involved.

As a fourth point, specific elements of attunement (or rapport) are important. Above all, it is essential for the involvement of the patient that you correctly attune to the use of language and avoid jargon. If you use 'fancy' words and jargon when talking to someone who uses simple language, you create distance between the two of you. This makes the patient feel less involved and they are more likely to behave passively.

Finally, the patient will become more involved if you pay attention to their personal considerations, concerns, and thoughts regarding their health problem. You can ask or respond to these issues if the patient brings them up in passing.

TAKING NOTES AND USING THE COMPUTER

During each consultation, you will likely want to make notes on paper or directly on the computer. During the diagnostic process in particular, you may need to process a considerable amount of information in the patient's file. However, you do not want this activity to disrupt your contact with the patient, or to interrupt or impede the patient's story. Frequent computer use at the beginning of the consultation also hampers building up the necessary relationship of trust due to the lack of eye contact and because you have fewer opportunities for attunement or modelling. It is well known that frequent computer usage during the consultation occurs at the expense of the content of the medical history and especially the patient's story (Margalit *et al.*, 2006; Silverman & Kinnersley, 2010).

Put Into Action: Taking Notes and Using the Computer

First of all, it is sensible to start your consultation without looking directly at the screen. Use the first one or two minutes to establish contact with the patient, make eye contact, and adjust your non-verbal and verbal modelling. In short, focus entirely on the patient in the first instance. In the next chapter, the importance of establishing the first contact will be discussed in more detail.

In order to make notes in the patient's computer file during the consultation, you'll need good typing skills. If you are not a proficient typist, it's better to make notes on paper. This can almost certainly be done without disrupting contact with the patient too much. You can also include some 'pauses for writing' during a conversation. At a suitable moment, tell the patient you want to take some notes. Break eye contact and preferably turn slightly away from the patient. This makes it clear that you have stopped listening for the moment and prevents the patient from continuing the conversation.

Finally, it is also possible to involve the computer in the conversation. This can be done, for example, by giving the patient insight into the 'physiotherapy analysis/diagnosis' at the end of the examination. By not merely explaining the analysis, but also letting the patient read on the computer screen what and how you have made a note of this in the file, you can enhance transparency and trust. There will probably also be other good opportunities to let the patient read what you have written in their file on the computer.

Summary

In this chapter, we have seen the physiotherapist at work in their role as a confidant. They provide structure during each consultation, from beginning to end, building and maintaining the relationship. The confidant also involves the patient in the consultation and keeps him involved by paying attention to aspects such as providing information, attuning to the patient's use of language and by asking personal questions. This enables them to work as a coach, communicative detective, and teacher. Using the computer can be a disruptive factor for the role of confidant, and therefore possibly also for the other roles. By dealing with the need to use the computer efficiently, however, this disruption can be prevented.

PART III

The Consultation

We now know the main points of a professional conversation and have established the basis for the conversation during the first consultation. Now the consultation will really take off. Within the consultation as a whole, the physiotherapy conversation is expanded in this part, with regard to the diagnostic as well as the therapeutic process. You can also see how the conversation usually develops and how you can guide this. Sticky, difficult, or complex situations and special or exceptional circumstances are dealt with in Part IV.

The chapters in this section follow the seven core tasks of the consultation. Because offering structure, building and maintaining the relationship, and involving and keeping the patient involved in all core tasks are relevant throughout, these aspects have already been discussed in Chapter 4.

This section begins with Chapter 5, in which the core task of 'initiating the consultation' is expanded. The 'gathering of information' with regard to the medical history and the patient's story is discussed in Chapter 6, and conducting the conversation during the 'physical examination' in Chapter 7. Chapter 8 then discusses the core tasks of 'explaining, making shared decisions, goal-setting, and making plans'. Chapter 9 focuses on the conversation during the 'treatment'.

'Concluding the consultation' often has its own implicit character. Still, it is good to think about this as well, and we shall do this in Chapter 10. The last chapter of this section, Chapter 11, discusses 'finishing the treatment episode'.

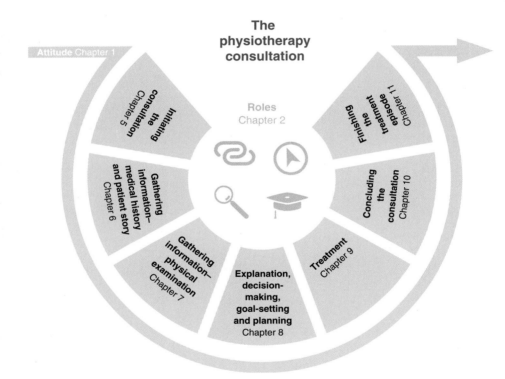

The physiotherapy consultation

Attitude Chapter 1

Initiating the consultation Chapter 5

Gathering information– medical history and patient story Chapter 6

Gathering information– physical examination Chapter 7

Explanation, decision-making, goal-setting and planning Chapter 8

Treatment Chapter 9

Concluding the consultation Chapter 10

Finishing the treatment episode Chapter 11

Roles Chapter 2

Initiating the Consultation

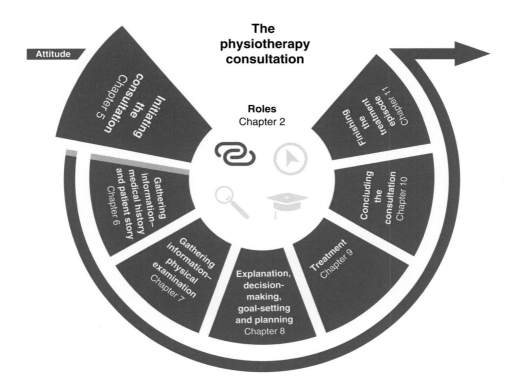

In the initial consultation, your very first contact with the patient is crucial. You are probably familiar with the saying, 'You never get a second chance to make a first impression'. This is also the case with a physiotherapy consultation. This first impression is, of course, important in order to build a relationship of trust with the patient. We already discussed the relationship of trust in the previous chapter, but because the first contact with the patient has some specific focal points, these are considered separately here. The patient relationship and the impression you make should never be far from your mind—you 'renew' the contact at the beginning of each subsequent consultation.

At the beginning of the consultation, you will bring up the 'agenda': What are everyone's expectations, what is the purpose of the consultation, and how can you best achieve this? Establishing the first contact and setting the agenda of the consultation with the patient corresponds with the role of the confidant. This immediately makes the work of the communicative detective (in core tasks 2, 3, and 4) and that of the coach and teacher (in core tasks 5, 6, and 7) a lot easier.

MAKING A POSITIVE FIRST IMPRESSION

The very first contact between the physiotherapist and the patient (e.g. in the waiting room) lays the foundation for the subsequent contact and the relationship of trust that you want to build with the patient. This means that the first contact has an influence on the course of the entire first consultation and on the following sessions.

It has been shown that the initial information people receive makes more of an impression than the information which follows. People tend to regard their first impression as the 'truth'. So a positive and warm first impression lingers. Moreover, a cool and distant first impression lingers even longer—several positive actions or contacts will be needed to 'erode' that to some extent (Demarais & White, 2007). In this way, a first impression acts as a kind of filter through which you look at the other person. People also tend to look for information which matches their filter. That is why someone will tend to ignore information that does not fit their first impression.

■ Filtering Errors

When processing information, certain 'filtering errors' often occur. A common mistake is that people tend to generalise the first impression they get of a person's personality or character and see it as applicable in all circumstances—not as a result of the situation in which they met the other person at the time. Furthermore, people tend to generalise someone's positive characteristics: a person with just one positive characteristic is seen to have many. This is also known as the 'halo effect'. So if someone has the (first) impression that the other person is friendly and patient, they are also more inclined to see them as skilled and competent. A generalisation of negative properties is known as the 'horn effect'.

By taking these filtering errors into account, you can make sure that the first impression you make on others is the impression you would like to make.

Put Into Action: Making a Positive First Impression

If you meet the following four (universal) social needs of people, there is a significant chance that you will make a positive impression (Demarais & White, 2007) on your patient by:
- showing appreciation;
- looking for a connection;
- lifting the mood;
- being informative.

You can show your appreciation by warmly welcoming or complimenting the other person. If you pay attention in a positive way to certain characteristics of the patient, they feel appreciated.

You also achieve this by focusing all your attention from the first moment on the other person and being interested in them. Connecting is done by making a 'connection', such as mentioning something that you and the patient have in common. For example, if you know a family member of the patient, you can bring this up and ask how they are doing. Or you might say something about the street where the patient lives, if you know it well. You can lift the mood by paying attention, smiling, and emphasising positive things (and not complaining or sighing, for example, about your slow computer or the weather). Finally, you can share information that the other person doesn't know and which may interest them. For example, you might explain what exactly it says on the GP's referral.

In subsequent consultations, renewing this contact is a focal point. In addition to the points discussed in Chapter 4 regarding building and maintaining the relationship of trust, it is good practice to use the first one or two minutes of each consultation to reconnect with your patient.

SETTING THE AGENDA FOR THE CONVERSATION

An effective consultation requires a good agenda. You want to bring up all the necessary themes, and you only have limited time to do so. It's a fairly tall order: you want the patient to tell their story, then analyse their health problem properly, give the patient good information, and link this adequately to the patient's request for help. In the role of confidant, you want to provide structure to achieve these goals, and for this you use a common agenda for the conversation. Remember, it is not only you who has a target and a method of working in mind; the patient probably does, too. It is good to realise this and to coordinate your expectations regarding the consultation. Research has shown that collaborating with the patient when setting the purpose and agenda of the consultation brings a number of benefits (Benedetti, 2013; Di Blasi et al., 2001; O'Keeffe et al., 2016). By doing so, the patient's involvement increases, they take more responsibility during the consultation, and they experience more satisfaction with regard to the consultation because their request for help is answered.

The agenda focuses on the goal of the consultation and discusses the method of achieving this goal, as well as how much time you have for this. This will help you to adequately fulfil your role as a communicative detective (or coach or teacher) while also achieving the goals you and the patient have in mind for the consultation. In order to structure the content of the themes during the first consultation, you use a thought structure as described in Chapter 3, such as 'screening' or 'taking a medical and patient history'. This kind of thought structure helps you to remember everything.

Put Into Action: Setting the Agenda for the Conversation

At the beginning of the diagnostic consultation, it is generally best to start by explaining how you would like to proceed during the consultation and to indicate that you would like to attune to the patient's expectations. A lot of patients find it difficult to clearly indicate what they actually expect from a consultation, so by bringing it up yourself and suggesting a proposal, you make it easier for most patients to share their ideas about it with you.

As an introduction, briefly explain your usual way of working (your specific working method or that of your practice or institution) and how you would like to approach it in this first consultation. Then ask the patient if they have had previous experience with physiotherapy and what they expect from the consultation. Say, for example: 'What do you hope to achieve with this consultation?' Finally, discuss your goals for the consultation and the appropriate way to achieve these goals. Indeed, your first questions could also be whether the patient has had previous experience of physiotherapy and what their expectations are, followed by an explanation of your own working method.

At the start of a consultation in the therapeutic process, your working method is not much different from that of a diagnostic consultation. Tell the patient what you would like to do and attune to them by finding out what their expectations are. After a few treatments, a certain routine may arise at the start of the consultations in the therapeutic process. That's fine. However, it is good to check regularly—for example, at the end of the consultation—whether the patient's expectations have been met and whether they would like to discuss other matters.

How much time you have available for the consultation should be relative to the goals of the conversation. If this is not the case, you have to make choices in consultation with the patient. After consultation with the patient, move some of your conversation to the next appointment. If you notice that certain points in the conversation take more time than you had anticipated, it is helpful to inform the patient of this at some point: 'Our conversation so far has taken more time than I expected, we're a little behind schedule'. Make an immediate proposal to deal with it. Don't hesitate to do so, because patients often don't feel responsible for the time available or are not as aware of the time. So remind them of this and make them co-responsible.

In Consultation

Attunement	Have you ever been to a physiotherapist before?
	(laughing) No, luckily I haven't!
Creating an agenda	(chuckles) Of course! I want to make sure this consultation meets your expectations. Shall I briefly tell you how I would like to approach this consultation or do you have specific expectations?
	Sure, just tell me what you would like to do.
	Well, at a first consultation, I usually listen carefully to what's bothering you. I'll do this by talking to you and physically examining you. If it's clear what's going on, I'll explain it to you. Together we will then look at the treatment possibilities and your own goals. We almost certainly won't have enough time for a treatment in this first consultation—that will come in the second consultation. Is this what you imagined this consultation would be or do you have other expectations?
	Well, that makes sense to me. I am, however, sorry that I won't be treated today.
Reflecting	Mmm, I can imagine. You're a little disappointed about that.
	Well, yes…it's too bad. A little bit, but I get it. Of course, you need to know what's wrong before you can start treatment.
Reflecting	A good analysis certainly forms the basis for a successful treatment. And usually
Explaining	the analysis takes so much time that there is no time left for actual treatment. I will probably manage to give you some advice, though.
	Oh, that's good. I'd specifically like to know what I can do about it myself.
Reflecting	Mmm, you would like to be able to do something about it yourself after this
Asking in-depth	consultation. What else do you hope to get from this consultation?
questions	*Well, that I know exactly what's going on and how to get rid of it.*
	That's understandable. Anything else?
	No.
Summarising	So at the end of this consultation, you want to know what's going on, how to deal with it, and know what your own role is?
	Yes, indeed.
Taking name and	Fine. If I can just put some of your administrative data into the computer, we can
address data	get going.
	Okay.
	What's your address? (turns to the computer screen)
	……
Asking an opening	Great, that's all in there (turns away from the computer and looks at the patient).
question	Tell me, what brings you here?

Summary

In this chapter, we have seen the confidant at work. In the role of confidant, you want to make a good first impression, so that further contact with the patient runs smoothly and a relationship of trust can be established. The confidant also provides structure by discussing the agenda of the conversation with the patient.

Gathering Information – Medical History and Patient Story

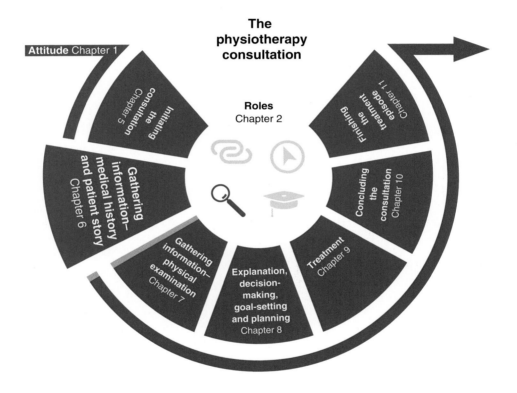

The conversation is now underway, and the relationship of trust between you and the patient is growing. You now start with the core task of 'gathering information'; in this task, you are active in the role of communicative detective. You and the patient start to examine what they have come for. You begin to look at the nature and seriousness of the health problem to analyse it. The analysis is only optimal if the patient 'co-analyses' and you therefore involve the patient as much as possible in this process. Thus, gathering information is not an activity in which the physiotherapist alone asks an overwhelming number of questions—the communication skills and techniques that you use as a physiotherapist have a much broader context and you are explicitly striving for patient participation.

For didactic reasons, in order to better understand and learn the core task of 'gathering information', we can divide this task into four components (not necessarily executed in this order):

- identifying the request for help;
- obtaining information;
- sharing information;
- establishing and explaining links.

While gathering information, both during the interview and the physical examination, you also form a picture of how the patient thinks about their health problem. These illness perceptions largely determine how the patient behaves in relation to their health problem. This behaviour can support but also hinder recovery. Exploring perceptions of illness is therefore given a separate section in this chapter.

The collection of information often continues during the physical examination. This chapter therefore concludes with transitioning from the interview to the physical examination.

IDENTIFYING THE REQUEST FOR HELP

The request for help is the (often implicit) question or purpose that the patient has in relation to their health problem. In other words: What do they hope and/or expect to achieve with physiotherapy? The patient's motivation for their visit sometimes seems very obvious. And yet it is actually less obvious than it seems. General requests for help, such as 'being treated for pain' and 'making a full recovery', are not necessarily the most important. Concerns about the duration of the health problem and its significance often play a role in patients' requests for help. Many patients also have the need to prevent the recurrence of their symptoms (McRae & Hancock, 2017).

Put Into Action: Identifying the Request for Help

Look for a suitable point to identify the request for help. Sometimes this is immediately after starting the conversation, after attuning to the patient's expectations about the consultation (see also Section 'Setting the agenda for conversation' in Chapter 5). Another suitable point can be when the patient has given you the necessary information about their symptoms and what they are facing—you now have a more rounded idea of what their health problem entails. Ask, for example: 'What do you expect physiotherapy to achieve?' or 'How can physiotherapy treatment or support help you with this?' Then listen carefully, reflecting on what the patient tells you and asking for further clarification where you think it is necessary.

Some patients find it difficult to articulate the request for help properly at the beginning of a physiotherapy consultation. Sometimes they only manage to do this in the course of the conversation. Others implicitly express their request for help 'wrapped up' in other statements. If the patient finds it difficult to express their request for help, help them by reflecting on their earlier statements and by using summaries.

The request for help can sometimes change in the course of the conversation—for example, because you are sharing information during the conversation. It is also possible that the request for help may change in the course of the treatment process. Keep this in mind. Evaluate or check regularly with the patient whether this is the case.

■ Dialogue Model

During the diagnostic or therapeutic process, it can be effective to use a 'dialogue model'. Especially when dealing with complex health problems, such as chronic pain, it may be wise to make use of it. This is a diagram or drawing (on paper or digital) used to structure the content of the conversation. The advantage of using such a model is that it supports the patient in their thinking (and analysis) and thereby stimulates the patient's participation in the consultation.

An example of a dialogue model that is well suited to the physiotherapy context is the 'equaliser' aid (Figure 6.1).

This model indicates that a health problem is the sum of all kinds of aspects and not just the result of a disorder. The extent to which an aspect plays a role is always displayed on the slider on the right. The number 1 shows that it plays an unimportant role; a 10 shows when the role is very important. Some aspects get a 1 or 2, some a 5, others an 8 or 9. The sum of all the 'scores' ultimately gives a description of the current health problem on which the treatment will focus. It more or less automatically conceptualises the patient's thinking about their health problem. It stimulates the patient to sufficiently consider their health problem in depth and breadth. It also helps in analysing causes and explaining the patient's symptoms.

GATHERING INFORMATION

During an initial interview, the gathering of information is pivotal. This information is medical, personal, and psychosocial in nature. As a communicative detective, you want to find information about the health problem, both medical and personal, in a targeted way. It's important you support the patient when they are telling you their personal story. Effective skills for gathering information are:

- listening;
- asking questions and in-depth questions;
- summarising;
- reflecting.

These four skills are briefly explained below. Keep in mind that you are constantly applying skills from the viewpoint of the role and attitude of the communicative detective. You will find an article detailing additional communication skills on Evolve.

Listening

Listening is a special skill. In the communication process, it is of course important to listen carefully and attentively. However logical this may seem, in practice it often goes wrong. First of all: paying full attention to the patient is not always easy. Many things distract us while we work. Attentive listening also means paying attention to the things the patient says and the words they use. After all, the phrases and words the patient uses say something about the thoughts they have. Moreover, listening carefully means that you are sensitive to the things the patient means to say, but does not say explicitly through their choice of words. In other words, try to read between the lines of the patient's statement. Reflecting this is very useful (see below). By listening attentively, the conversation reaches a 'higher level of communication'. Finally, listening also lets the patient know that you have heard and understood them. So you not only have to be attentive, but also show this by looking at the other person, nodding and/or saying 'Hmmm' at certain points, using facial expressions or giving signals with other parts of the body, reflecting, having an 'open' posture, and using silences.

Asking Questions and In-Depth Questions

Questions can stimulate the patient to dig deeper into the topic or to add themes to the conversation. In other words: questions can be intended to dig deeper and find out more. In this way, you can 'deepen' the conversation by asking more about an existing theme or subject; for example, 'How would you describe that feeling?' or 'What do you think is happening to your knee?' If you want to broaden your question, you introduce a new conversation topic, such as: 'To what extent do you think

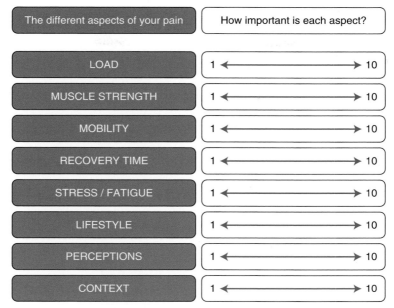

Figure 6.1 Dialogue model: equaliser aid.

stress or fatigue plays a role?' or 'How do your family members deal with the fact that you have these problems?' Open questions are especially suitable to deepen and broaden the conversation.

Finally, you can steer the conversation in a certain direction by asking questions. In Chapter 4 Section "Providing structure", this is referred to as 'directive questioning' and explained as a concept. What you actually do with directive questioning is to influence the direction in which someone thinks. By taking advantage of this, you can benefit from asking an open question and at the same time steering the direction of the conversation.

Summarising

Summarising is an extremely useful skill for bringing structure to the conversation. You list the patient's statements and show how they all relate to each other. This not only creates clarity and an overview for the patient, but also for yourself. You can also check whether you have understood the patient correctly. Furthermore, it is often useful to summarise when you want to conclude an important theme in the conversation and move on to the next.

Reflecting

Reflecting is giving back to the patient what they said or what you think they meant to say. The effect is that the patient notices that you have been listening. Moreover, when they hear their own utterance (in other words or otherwise), they reflect upon it further and are stimulated to carry on talking about it, for example, by providing further information.

To reflect your patient adequately, you need empathy (see also Section "Attitude skills" in Chapter 1). Empathy means that you look at, hear, and sense the world from the patient's frame of reference, as if you were the patient. By reflecting, you help the patient to put into words what they want to say: you reflect their thoughts and feelings. Reflecting has a powerful positive effect on the relationship with your patient.

You can give reflections in the form of a question. For example, you may say: 'I gather from what you've told me that you're very worried, am I right?' It is also possible to give reflections without a question mark, such as: 'You're sick of it and you'd like to do it differently'. Of course, your tone of voice throughout has to be mild and empathic. An advantage of this technique is that the patient may feel more like they have said it themselves, which makes them think about themselves in more depth. For the patient, your reflection is like listening to an echo of themselves, but with a deeper content. The effect is that the patient wonders (and speculates) whether this is indeed what they intended and corrects and/or supplements this. It deepens the patient's' story. The patient also takes note of the fact that you are making an effort to understand and listen to them.

Put Into Action: Gathering Information

You use the skills of listening, asking questions, summarising, and reflecting in the role of the communicative detective to obtain information. There are a few points of interest here.

During the core task of 'gathering information', you introduce several subjects. This can sometimes be tricky—for example, if you find it difficult to broach a particular subject, or if you notice that the patient finds it difficult to talk about a certain topic. A good opening question can then help. Opening questions are those that address specific themes in a conversation for the first time. Opening questions relate to, for example, psychosocial themes such as stress, one's own beliefs, lifestyle, social influence, range of motion, and so on. A 'Question Lexicon' is available on Evolve, with question phrases that you can use when broaching a 'new' conversation topic. You may not find all the questions easy to work with, but the Question Lexicon is a resource that you can use to your own advantage; over time, you will probably develop a question lexicon of your own.

Sometimes a patient does not react in a good way when you ask a lot of open questions; they don't understand what you mean or they find it difficult to react. In this case, give your question a little more direction. For example, if the patient does not respond well to a question such as 'What other things are aggravating your problem?', continue with 'Which things, at work, for example, make your symptoms worse?' or 'In what sense does your work worsen your problem?' Sometimes this can also be done in two steps: first ask a closed question, then an open question. For example: 'Are your complaints aggravated by your work?' and if the patient answers in the affirmative: 'How exactly?'

If a conversation contains too many questions, there is a chance that the patient will experience it as an 'interrogation'. This puts the relationship of trust in jeopardy. It is important to regularly alternate your questions with reflections during the conversation. Reflecting makes the patient feel understood and supported, and the conversation becomes more of a dialogue. An additional advantage is that your reflections help the patient to express themselves, exploring what they mean and digging deeper, which is useful for the communicative detective. The adequate use of reflections during a conversation does require some practice—it is not an easy skill.

▪ Normalising

Although the patient may find it difficult to exchange ideas with you about certain topics, there is no need to panic about addressing a potentially tricky theme. Acting too cautiously and carefully will only add to the 'emotional load', making the conversation difficult and uncomfortable, both for you and for the patient. By 'normalising' a topic in this respect, you help yourself and the patient. Normalising means that you do not deal differently with 'difficult' themes than with 'easier' themes. So if, for example, you are talking to the patient about possible causes for their health problem, you can explore what role physical stress and, in a similar way, distress plays in their lives.

Another aspect worth considering is if you feel reluctance to discuss a certain topic with your patient. In this case, it's good to talk to yourself about this. Are you in doubt whether such a theme can actually play a role in the issue? Do you differ in age from the patient and may this be holding you back? Do you think the patient doesn't expect some issues to be addressed by a physiotherapist? Ask yourself where your hesitation comes from and work on it so that it diminishes.

By summarising several times while taking the medical history, you organise the information up to that moment. It is possible to link a 'pause for writing' to these moments of summarising, in which you take a moment to write down the most important information and the patient is given some time to reflect.

When obtaining information, your own choice of words is important. You may have already experienced that a small change in the way you formulate something makes a big difference: the question suddenly doesn't sound as good as it did before. Your intonation and your expression are also very important. Sensitivity to your own use of words, your intonation, and your non-verbal behaviour and body language helps you to obtain more reliable information and gives you a good picture of the patient's perceptions more quickly.

Finally, it is important to pay attention to the patient's choice of words, intonation, and non-verbal expression. These say a lot about the patient's perceptions. And these perceptions, in turn, (partly) determine the way in which they behave.

SHARING INFORMATION

People tend to look for cause-effect relationships. After all, we assume that there are connections between the things we see and what we experience. For example, a patient who suffers back pain immediately after doing something that, in their opinion, causes back pain will tend to think that their back pain was caused by this activity, even if this is not at all the case. Because people make conclusions from 'logical' connections' such as these, it is very useful to first share some information with the patient on some of the topics you want to address in your consultation. As a detective, you are being communicative by informing the patient about a specific subject so that they understand why it is relevant to discuss it and also so they know what they need to think about. This allows them to participate better in the analysis of their own health problem and become more open to addressing certain themes in the conversation, such as psychosocial aspects of the situation. Share the exact information that the patient needs to participate fully in the process of analysis of their health problem: not too little, but not too much either. The appropriate amount will vary from patient to patient, depending on their prior knowledge.

Themes which require the patient to be given prior information are, for example, the connection between health problems and stress, lifestyle, lack of exercise, being overweight, and one's own beliefs. Many patients are often not aware of these connections or only insufficiently so. If they gain insight into these themes, they are then better able to discover possible connections by themselves. So if you explain to someone how stress can arise and how this can contribute to certain injuries, they may become motivated to think about that consciously. Understanding the type of strain that can lead to an injury to a part of the body also helps the patient to determine whether they may have overexerted themselves for a period of time.

Put Into Action: Sharing Information

A lot of information about our health is complicated. It is important to simplify complex information and use, for example, comparisons or metaphors. It is more important that the patient understands some of the issue rather than nothing, even if it is a simplification (as in a metaphor). A step-by-step plan for sharing information is: prompt – share – prompt.

- **Prompt:** Explore what the patient already knows and ask permission to provide (additional) information.

    By first ascertaining the patient's prior knowledge, you activate their brain. This creates fertile ground for what follows. You do this by asking a question about it. Often, you already have an idea of what the patient knows about a specific subject. Summarise this first and then check whether the patient may know more about it. Then ask the patient for permission to give them additional information.

- **Share:** Share the information.
  If you know what the patient has knowledge of, you can connect to it to the new knowledge in exactly the right area.
- **Prompt:** Ascertain if the patient understands and ask them what this means to them.
  It is, of course, necessary for the patient to apply the knowledge you've just provided. Therefore, first check that the patient has understood and then ask them: 'What does this information mean to you?' or 'If I tell you like this, can you do something with it? What exactly?'

A good example in which you can use this step-by-step plan during the diagnostic process is in determining the connection between the health problem and stress. If you first prompt the patient to tell you what they know about the connection between stress and their 'type' of health problem, and then share information (after permission) about this connection with the patient, it becomes considerably easier to discuss this topic with the patient and to analyse the role stress plays. If you don't do this, the patient may respond negatively to your questions about stress.

Sharing information with the patient is not always easy—for example, if the information itself is complicated. In the Section "Giving advice" in Chapter 9, we will go into more detail on how you can do this effectively with health information and education.

Asking Permission

You ask for permission at all sorts of times during the conversation with the patient. Typical of these moments is that you want to give information or advice to the patient and you want the patient to be open to what you have to say.

It may seem a little strange that you must ask permission at these moments; you may think something like 'It's logical that the patient gives permission for that—that's what they do'. It is still beneficial to do so consciously.

By asking for *explicit* permission at these moments, you emphasise the autonomy of the patient. You also *implicitly* give the signal that the patient's opinion matters and that you want to work *with* them and not be in charge of them. If the patient then gives you permission, they are (more) open to what you have to say.

Asking permission is therefore a method in which you also choose your approach because of the implicit aspects of your message, not just because of your explicit literal message (von Thun, 1981).

ESTABLISHING AND EXPLAINING LINKS

Analysing the patient's health problem automatically leads to making all kinds of connections or links, such as between the signs and symptoms on the one hand and the disorder or syndrome on the other hand, or between cause and effect, between patient behaviour and the trajectory of the health problem, or between the load and the load capacity. Making connections is part of the clinical reasoning process. This book is based on the principle that the patient is involved as much as possible in the analysis of their health problem. This is exactly why the physiotherapist is communicative: they present the connections they think they see to the patient and try to give explanations. Together with the patient, they also try to establish a connection with the request for help and discuss the possibilities and impossibilities.

Put Into Action: Establishing and Explaining Links

Offering and explaining those connections you think you see presents a number of focal points. First of all, the certainty of a link may vary. Sometimes you feel very certain about something; sometimes it's only one of the possibilities. The degree of certainty is reflected in the way you discuss the relationship with the patient, verbally and non-verbally.

Secondly, some factors that are relevant to the health problem lie well within your field of expertise (the physiotherapy domain) while others are at the margin or beyond it. Your main area of expertise, for example, is establishing the link between a pinching and gripping movement and the development of a tennis elbow. At the margin of your field, for example, is *determining* the connection between stress and the health problem. Researching why the patient experiences stress at work lies beyond your area of expertise. A rule of thumb is that the degree of physiotherapy expertise you have deployed determines how confidently you present the connection you think you see to the patient. The less physiotherapy expertise, the lower the certainty will probably be.

Furthermore, knowledge is often needed to make connections. So before you present a presumed connection to the patient, you have to determine whether they have sufficient knowledge to analyse this. If not, an explanation is required. The step-by-step plan from the previous section, 'prompt – share – prompt', is useful here.

Finally, you must selectively present those links that are important in the context of the patient's request for help or which you believe will help the patient's insight into the illness (the patient's illness perceptions).

■ Infographic

A tool that can be useful in collecting and organising information about the health problem is the dialogue model: the infographic. In the infographic, you put together all relevant information about the patient's health problem. It consists of an empty sheet of paper, divided into four sections. Figure 6.2 shows a completed example. Such a tool is particularly useful when dealing with complex health problems.

Each box is a separate section, with information on, respectively:
- signs and symptoms, complaints, disabilities;
- causes, origin, development, barriers to recovery;
- conclusion, analysis, personal goals;
- plan, actions and strategy.

The four sections are filled with relevant information while taking the medical history and while doing the physical examination. The therapist can do this, but so can the patient. The infographic thus takes shape through collaboration between the two. It is therefore important that both the patient and the therapist get to see the paper with the infographic.

Connections between factors are indicated by arrows.

The infographic takes shape during the investigation. This helps to figure out the patient's health problem while at the same time giving the patient insight.

The Analysis

Gathering information means looking for relevant information along with the patient. By first sharing specific information with your patient at certain times, you make the patient a little 'wiser', so that they can participate more actively in the analysis of their own health problem. Often, they will also be better able to answer your questions and look for relevant information themselves.

In this way, you facilitate your collaboration with the patient, something you are striving for during the analysis of the health problem. If the patient participates as far as possible within their abilities, the result is a broader and deeper analysis, which is therefore more complete. By paying attention to your own language and that of the patient, and to non-verbal communication as well, the final analysis becomes even stronger. By using good question formulations, you stimulate the patient to express their own thoughts and feelings. The way the patient then expresses their thoughts can say a lot about how they think about their health problem or their illness perceptions.

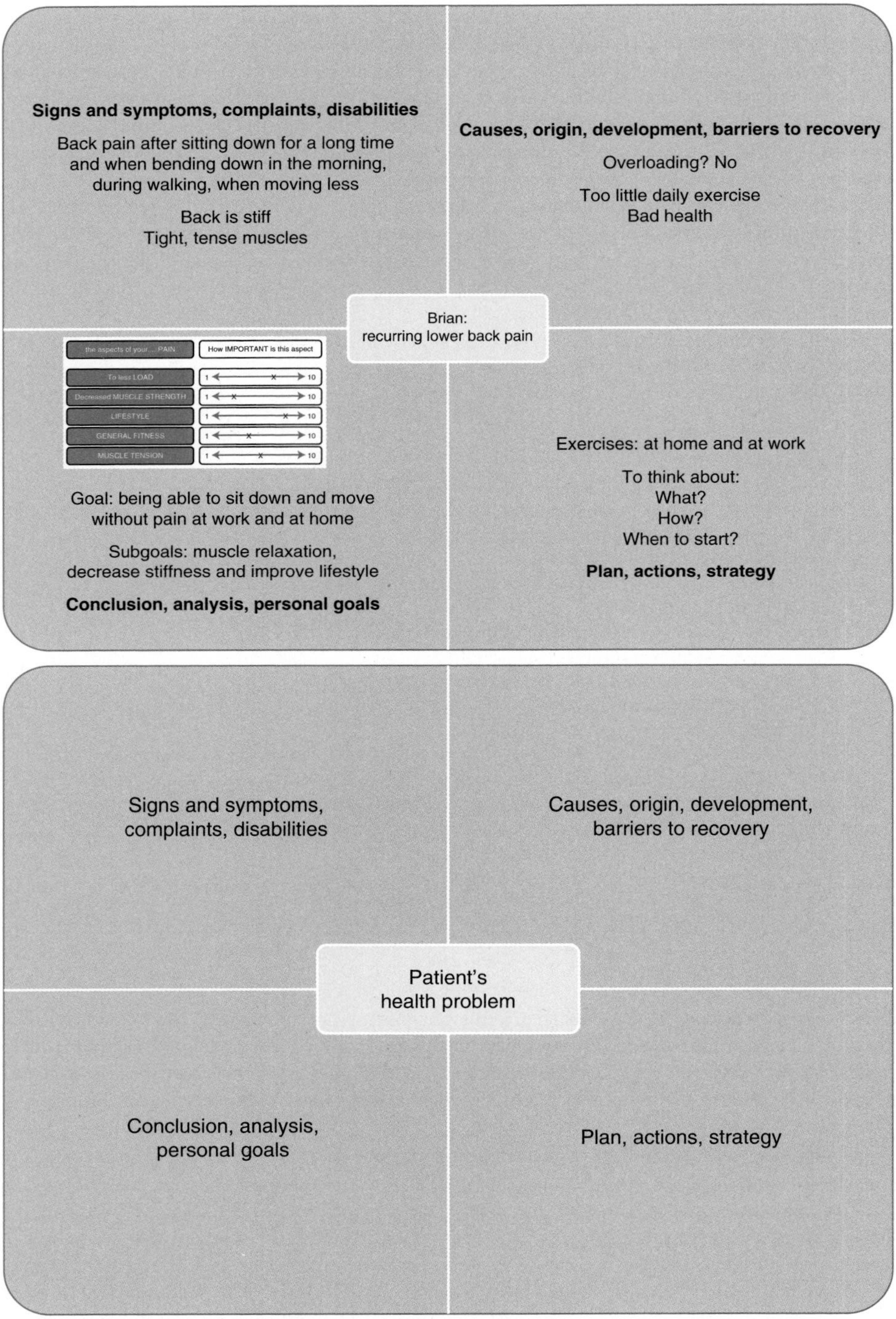

Signs and symptoms, complaints, disabilities

Back pain after sitting down for a long time
and when bending down in the morning,
during walking, when moving less

Back is stiff
Tight, tense muscles

Causes, origin, development, barriers to recovery

Overloading? No

Too little daily exercise
Bad health

Brian:
recurring lower back pain

the impacts of your ....PAIN	How IMPORTANT is this aspect
To less LOAD	1 ←——x——→ 10
Decreased MUSCLE STRENGTH	1 ←—x——→ 10
LIFESTYLE	1 ←———x—→ 10
GENERAL FITNESS	1 ←——x——→ 10
MUSCLE TENSION	1 ←——x——→ 10

Goal: being able to sit down and move
without pain at work and at home

Subgoals: muscle relaxation,
decrease stiffness and improve lifestyle

Conclusion, analysis, personal goals

Exercises: at home and at work

To think about:
What?
How?
When to start?

Plan, actions, strategy

Signs and symptoms,
complaints, disabilities

Causes, origin, development,
barriers to recovery

Patient's
health problem

Conclusion, analysis,
personal goals

Plan, actions, strategy

Figure 6.2 Example of a patient infographic.

EXPLORING ILLNESS PERCEPTIONS

While gathering information, the patient reveals all kinds of thoughts and ideas about their health problem. These thoughts and ideas are called 'illness perceptions' or 'illness beliefs'. If you have a good picture of the patient's illness perceptions, you can, among other things, make a better decision about the patient's health behaviour and recovery.

The concept of illness perceptions is described by Leventhal in the Common Sense Model of Self-Regulation (Cameron & Leventhal, 2003). This model describes the thoughts and feelings that patients have about what exactly is going on, how long complaints can last, what the cause may be, how it can be solved, and by whom. A patient reacts to a health-threatening stimulus such as pain or stiffness both cognitively and emotionally, developing certain perceptions as a result. These perceptions strongly guide the behaviour they will exhibit, behaviour with which the patient wants to remove the health-threatening stimulus. The Common Sense Model of Self-Regulation has been researched extensively. Considerable evidence indicates that the cognitive dimension in particular (usually called illness perceptions) guides a person's behaviour—in other words, how they act is affected by the thoughts a person has about their 'illness' (Hagger & Orbell, 2003). Leventhal has described (Cameron & Leventhal, 2003) the following related illness perceptions for the cognitive dimension:

- the identity (what's going on? what is it?);
- the cause (what's the cause?);
- the timeline (how long will it take?);
- the consequences (what are the consequences?);
- the controllability and curability (how can I get it under control and how can I recover?).

In practice, it is perplexing that patients always question themselves about the above, but often subconsciously. Because of this, they are regularly unable to adequately answer the physiotherapist's questions about their illness perceptions. Nevertheless, all patients have formed 'pre-conscious' ideas and often act according to these ideas. This behaviour can promote or impede recovery. For example, if a patient thinks that their back pain will last a long time because they think of the pain as serious, they will experience a lot of negative effects which they think are beyond their control; this often leads to the patient becoming passive. In the end, it is therefore very possible that these perceptions form an obstacle to recovery and regaining normal functional movement (Foster et al., 2008; Hagger & Orbell, 2003).

The above makes it clear that it is crucial to get an idea of the patient's illness perceptions and to determine whether these are potentially impeding or conducive to recovery. Note that the fifth domain of the model, controllability and curability, is strongly related to the patient's request for help.

Although the cognitive dimension in particular has been proven to guide the patient's behaviour, it is certainly useful to get to know the patient's feelings about their health problem. Although this emotional dimension is less well elaborated in the Common Sense model, it also strongly influences the (illness) behaviour of the patient.

Put Into Action: Exploring Illness Perceptions

Exploring illness perceptions is something you do throughout the consultation—it is not reserved for a certain part of the consultation.

The first requirement for finding out about the patient's illness perceptions is 'excellent' listening. By listening carefully to what the patient says and what they intend to say, you can often get a good idea of how they think and feel about their health problem. Linking to what they say, the patient's line of thinking comes up for discussion in a very natural way. In every statement in the consultation, often right from the start, you can hear the patient's thoughts and feelings. Both by listening to what they state explicitly and also by 'reading between the lines', one hears the patient say something about their views on their health problem, how they interpret their pain, what it means to them, and how they deal with it. For example, if the patient says, 'I first tried to get some relief from it with a warm compress and by putting less strain on it', then a possible interpretation of this is that the patient thinks their muscles are very tense and that warmth and rest are a good solution for this. You can then reflect this statement to the patient to test this interpretation.

■ Language and Illness Perceptions

It can be difficult to articulate things you feel or think accurately and convey them to the person you are talking to. The process in which the patient (speaker) expresses their thoughts or feelings and the physiotherapist (listener) tries to understand this is shown in Figure 6.3. Errors arise in this process. You can reduce this by reflecting as a physiotherapist, i.e. presenting to the patient what you think they meant and thereby testing whether you have understood it correctly (the fourth arrow). In this way, you also help the patient by allowing them to hear their own statement, expressed in an alternative way, and then to adjust or clarify it. This creates an increasingly incisive idea of what the patient means, both for the patient and for you as a physiotherapist.

Sometimes excellent listening fails to provide a good picture of a situation. You then have to ask explicitly what the patient thinks about their health problem. The formulation of the question and the way you ask it are crucial. You don't want the patient, because of the implicit message in your question, to get the idea that you don't know what's wrong with them and that is why you are asking that question. That could happen if you ask, 'Do you yourself have any idea what's going on?' Instead, good questions to start the discussion about the patient's illness perceptions include 'What do you think is going on?' or, starting at the cause, 'Have you been able to come up with a cause for your complaints?' or, more extensively, 'You have already told me a lot, which gives me a fairly good idea of what is going on. Before I share that with you, I wonder how you feel about it. What do you think is going on?'

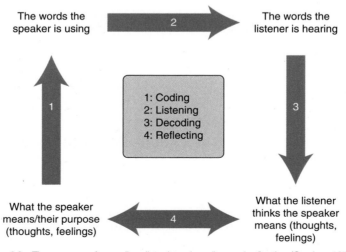

Figure 6.3 The process of encoding, listening, decoding and reflecting (Gordon, 1977).

In addition to the cognitive dimension, it is useful to discuss the patient's feelings and emotions in relation to their health problem. Think of how the patient worries about pain or recovery, or feels tense, despondent, sad, sceptical, etc. After the patient has articulated their idea of what is going on or could be going on, you could ask them, for example, 'What effect does that have on you?' or 'What does that do to your mood if you think it won't pass?'

In the Question Lexicon, available on Evolve, you will find more examples of questions on illness perceptions.

Throughout the conversation, you explore the patient's illness perceptions from the role of communicative detective. In the end, you then summarise your interpretations of the patient's illness perceptions. You do this not only to test whether you have understood it all correctly, but also to share your analysis with the patient and thus include them in your clinical reasoning process. What do the patient's perceptions mean for their behaviour and possibly for their health problem?

The example below clearly shows that by combining reflections and questions, the patient and the physiotherapist make more progress in their analysis than by asking questions alone. Above all, they gain more clarity about the patient's illness perceptions.

In Consultation

	A lot of everyday movements don't really bother me, but sometimes it hits me all of a sudden. It's like a nerve or something. If that pain then carries on, it really drives me crazy.
Reflecting	The pain is really intense.
	Yes, the pain is so intense I just feel like dying. My whole shoulder then hurts intensely and I can't do anything with it for a while. For a few minutes, I'm totally out of it. Sometimes I just feel like crying.
Reflecting	That intense sudden pain then just takes over.
	At these moments, I often think: this can't be good, there must be something really serious going on.
	And you think 'something serious' is a nerve?
	Well, I don't know. It feels so intense, more like something's really damaged, broken or something.
Reflecting	Mmm, the severe pain makes you think it's a serious injury.
Asking in-depth questions	Understandable. At what sort of times does it bother you this much?
	Yes, well, um, with sudden movements, it's often. So if I move more quickly or make an unexpected movement, it usually hits me.
Asking in-depth questions	To what extent does the type of movement you make with your arm affect you?
	Well, turning round is certainly annoying, like when I'm putting on my coat. And nothing much else affects it, I guess. Every sudden movement: forwards, sideways, upwards, I feel it every time.
Same conversation without reflections, with (open) questions	*A lot of everyday movements don't really bother me, but sometimes it hits me all of a sudden. It's like a nerve or something. If that pain then carries on, it really drives me crazy.*
Opening question	At what sort of times does it bother you this much?
	Yes, well, um, with sudden movements, it's often. So if I move more quickly or make an unexpected movement, it usually hits me.
Asking in-depth questions	Does the type of movement you make with your arm make a difference? I mean, in which direction?
	Well, turning round is certainly annoying, like when I'm putting on my coat. And nothing much else affects it, I guess. Every sudden movement: forwards, sideways, upwards, I feel it every time.

MONITORING THE REQUEST FOR HELP

Exploring the patient's request for help is part of core tasks 2, 3, and 4 (also see Section "Identifying the request for help" in Chapter 6). Because you regularly share information with the patient during further consultation, it is possible that the patient may reformulate their request for help. This is logical and also good. Many patients find it difficult to articulate their request for help properly and smoothly, so oftentimes, this is more or less done in chunks during the course of the consultation. Precisely because you involve and keep the patient involved during the consultation, they often manage to improve in formulating their request for help. During the consultation, the patient may also need to reformulate their request for help because it appears that certain goals they have in mind are not (or no longer) achievable.

If, in spite of everything, the patient's request for help is not sufficiently clear at the end of the interview or physical examination, bring this up and discuss with the patient what they would like to achieve and what they expect from a physiotherapy examination and/or treatment. Say, for example, 'At the beginning of the conversation, we talked about what you expect from a possible course of physiotherapy treatment. In the meantime, you have gained some insight into what is going on, and what is and is not feasible. How does that affect your expectations?'

USE OF CLINIMETRICS DURING THE CONSULTATION

Clinimetrics has become an indispensable part of today's care. It helps the communicative detective to arrive at a sharper analysis and makes the care needed much more clear. Sometimes, however, clinimetrics seems to be so central in the care process that it actually starts to pose a danger to the quality of physiotherapy care. The relationship with the patient becomes dominated by the use of clinimetrics and jeopardises your role as a confidant.

Some suggestions for communication during the use of clinimetrics (in the form of questionnaires) include:

- Introduce the questionnaire by indicating that you want to use it and say why. Say, for example, 'In order to get a picture of your shoulder complaints which is as objective as possible, I would like to do a short questionnaire with you. Are you familiar with this?' or 'In order to determine how much you are recovering (or progressing in terms of your performance), I would like to use a questionnaire. Are you familiar with this?'
- Then indicate the most important practical characteristics of the questionnaire, such as the number of questions, what the questions are mainly about, and how you want to conduct the questionnaire (on site, online, etc.). Think carefully about your explanation because it may influence your measurement.
- Give the patient a chance to ask questions. Listen, reflect, ask, and summarise.
- Provide brief and clear feedback on the results from the questionnaire so that the patient is well aware of the findings, avoid technical concepts relating to scores/rates, and keep a close eye on the main and side issues.

TRANSITION FROM HISTORY-TAKING TO PHYSICAL EXAMINATION

Before you start the next core task, the physical examination, it is necessary to give a summary of the information from the current core task. In this summary, present your interpretations and analysis of the patient's health problem one more time. Briefly list the hypotheses you have about the patient's health problem and their request for help. In the physical examination, you want to test your analysis, or parts of it, further. By concluding with what you want to test in the examination, you take the patient into the analysis process and create a smooth transition from the interview to the physical examination.

In Consultation

Opening question	What brings you here?
	Well, I've been having a lot of trouble with my right thigh for a couple of weeks now. It's at the back, I believe it's called my hamstring. It feels like a kind of cramp, but it also hurts. And it just won't go away, won't improve. It also doesn't get much worse, by the way, but annoyingly it doesn't go away.
Explore request for help	That's certainly where your hamstring is. With what sort of movements does it bother you?
	Well, it bothers me most when I'm exercising. I play hockey and then it really bothers me. And I feel it especially in the beginning. Once I'm warm and busy exercising and so on, I don't really feel it anymore. Only after training or competition, when I have cooled down again, I feel the pain quite strong again. So it seems to have something to do with whether the muscle is warmed up or not. And the day after exercising, it often bothers me more. Then I feel it when I go cycling and also when simply walking.
Asking in-depth questions	Are there any other times it bothers you?
	Well, I feel it at all sorts of times, but I can usually do everything. Up till now I've also continued exercising. That's okay, but it mustn't get any worse—I think I'd do less exercise then. That's what I'm wondering, maybe I should stop exercising, temporarily.
Reflecting	You are wondering if you will have a better recovery if you stop exercising for a while. I will get back to you on that as soon as it's clear what's going on. All right?
	Mmm, fine.
Asking in-depth questions	What can you do to trigger that annoying feeling in your leg?
	That cramping pain always comes when I bend over with my knees straight.
Opening question Summary Asking in-depth questions	Mmm, so you're experiencing a cramping pain in the back of your right leg which gets worse after exercise and you trigger it when you stretch your hamstring. To what extent do you have other complaints?
	I don't notice anything else, it's just the pain in my hamstring.
Opening question	Apart from the area around your hamstring, have you noticed anything?
	Um, no, I don't think so. What sort of things should I be thinking about?
Asking in-depth question Clarification	You may have noticed things that are unusual for you, somewhere else in your body and which you do not associate with this injury.
	Um, no. No, not that I can remember.
	Sensitivity or pain, stiffness maybe somewhere else in your leg, your groin, buttocks and pelvis, your back?
	No.
Opening question	Good. I would now like to look more closely at what's causing it. Do you have any ideas about that?
	Well, I've been thinking about that myself, but I haven't been able to figure out why it's happening. That pain, it actually came suddenly.
Reflection Sharing information	So the problem seems to have arisen spontaneously. It seems to me that we need to investigate this further. Maybe we can find a cause and with that an explanation for your problem, so that we can make sure that you will recover and that it will not come back.
	Yes, that would be nice if we could.
Sharing information Gathering information	It could be that a sudden increase in your physical stress has caused you to suffer from these problems. Or a change in the type of stress, for example by starting with certain strengthening exercises or the like. If you look back at the last two months, could there have been any change with regard to your physical stress?
	Well, sort of, I guess. I went back to hockey five weeks ago after the summer holidays. And before that I didn't play hockey for a year because I had started my studies, and because of the travelling I couldn't keep playing hockey.

Continued

In Consultation—cont'd

Asking in-depth questions	Ah, that certainly seems relevant. So you haven't played hockey for a year?
	Yes, over a year, almost a year and a half.
	And what did you do for exercise that year?
	Well, since I wanted to keep exercising, I went running. I did that two or three times a week. Usually something between five and eight kilometres.
Asking in-depth questions	When you started playing hockey again in August/September, how did you build up your training?
	(laughing) Actually, no. I mean, I just started as if I had never stopped. Had a lot of muscle ache in the first two weeks, too, I'm thinking now! In my buttocks, my back, and my legs. Oh, that was so awful, I looked really decrepit sometimes, I was so stiff! And then slowly the hamstring got worse. The rest of the muscle ache disappeared, but that stayed. And is still there.
Sharing information	It's good we're talking about this. This might indeed explain how it started.
Making/explaining links	In the period you weren't playing hockey, you put a completely different stress on your hamstring. Then you started playing hockey and you may not have given your muscles, and your hamstrings in particular, enough time to get used to this stress. And hockey and five kilometres of running do very different things to your body!
	So I probably overloaded my hamstring because I switched too quickly from running to hockey, and now my right hamstring is still affected. Doesn't that fix itself then, and why don't I have it on my left leg?
Asking permission	Those are two good questions. May I give you my answer to your first question?
	(nods)
Sharing information	It could well be that your current stress, and especially playing hockey, is
Closed question	preventing recovery. Or maybe your hamstring isn't strong enough, which is why you are still in pain. In that context, it is also interesting that you are suffering on the right and not on the left. Maybe the right one is not as strong. Or it could be that you are putting a much heavier load on the right than on the left. Can you comment on this: Is there a difference in the stress between the left and the right in your opinion?
	Um, I find that tricky. I don't think I put more stress on the right than on the left or vice versa.
Sharing information	Mmm, what's known about hockey is that to hit the ball, you bend down,
Asking in-depth question	putting your weight onto one leg, with the hamstring of that leg taking almost all the strain. Which stroke do you think is your favourite?
	My backhand. I play left winger and my backhand is my strongest stroke anyway. So I hit these a lot, also a lot more often when training.
Making links	Is it true that when you hit a backhand, you stand bent over with your
Closed question	weight on your right leg?
	Yes, that's right, and I'll move my left leg backwards.
Making/explaining links	Then that might well be the explanation. You therefore put far more strain on the hamstring of your right leg because you hit a backhand much more often. And with that you will obviously continue to stress your right hamstring too much, and your problem won't go away.
	Oh, of course. Boy, yes, well, that's pretty obvious. So the solution is to use my backhand less often for the time being?
	Yes, probably, yes. Besides that, you need to do other things. When I examine you in a minute, I'm also going to look at the muscle strength of your thighs, your flexibility, and a number of other things. Because, of course, this may not be the whole picture.

For comparison, we can go through the conversation with the same patient one more time. The therapist asks different questions (different directive questions), steers the conversation (possibly subconsciously) in a certain direction through their use of specific words, and is clearly less 'communicative'.

In Consultation

Opening question	What complaint do you have?
	I have some kind of cramp on the back of my thigh. It's painful, but fortunately not very painful.
Asking in-depth questions	Can you point it out?
	Yes, right here.
Asking in-depth questions	Mmm. And when does that bother you?
	Especially when I am doing exercise, I play hockey. Particularly at the start of a training session or game. Once I'm warm, I often don't feel it anymore. And after training or a competition, once I have cooled down again, I usually feel it very badly.
Asking in-depth questions	Do you only suffer during and immediately after hockey?
	Yes, as a matter of fact, I do.
Asking in-depth questions	Does bending down while keeping your legs straight hurt even when you're not exercising?
	Mmm, that's hard to say. Now, my ...
Asking in-depth questions	Stretch from your back, so to speak (demonstrating).
	Uh, yes, I can feel it.
Opening question	Have you ever had these complaints before?
	No.
Opening question	Do you have any other injuries at the moment?
	No, I have no complaints.
Asking in-depth questions	Or have you had any injuries in the past year?
	No, I haven't.
Opening question	How did it happen, did something happen?
	No, not that I know of.
Asking in-depth questions	Have you done things differently to usual? More, or indeed less, hockey playing?
	Well, that could be. I didn't play hockey at all last season.
Asking in-depth question	Right, so you started exercising again just after the summer?
	Yes, that's right.
Sharing information	Mmm, then of course, it's not that strange. Hamstring injuries are common among hockey players. So you have strained yourself. That means that you shouldn't put any stress on it, so no hockey for a while.
	Oh, really? But it surely can't be all that bad. I mean, I trained the day before yesterday. Then it does bother me, but it comes right again.
Giving advice	No, I don't think that's wise. You really shouldn't put so much strain on your hamstring, only then will it recover.
	But can't I do some light exercise and things that put less strain on my muscle?
Giving advice	Well, maybe some cycling, or maybe some running.
	Oh, so that is something at least!

In this last example, the physiotherapist's advice leads to an analysis that ends up being too narrow. You might say they do all the work themselves. Because of their closed questions, they also 'funnel' their analysis early on in the conversation. And they learn virtually nothing about the patient's thoughts and ideas. In addition, the patient also acquires virtually no insight during the interview. If the physiotherapist then tells the patient what is going on and what the solution is, the patient will feel overwhelmed much more quickly and dissonance (or friction) may even arise in the relationship between the patient and the physiotherapist. This also increases the chance that the patient will not see exactly what is going on and why the solution 'advised' by the physiotherapist is (or could be) the right one.

Summary

In this chapter, we've seen the communicative detective at work. During the interview, you try to find out what the patient's request for help is and gather information in order to be able to appropriately analyse the health problem. You take the patient into the process as a collaborative partner by not only asking them questions, but also by explaining things during the analysis so that they are also able to analyse the situation with this knowledge. In this explanation, you use three steps: prompt – share – prompt. Wherever possible, in the role of communicative detective, you look at links and connections and discuss these with the patient. The patient's illness perceptions play a role in this process. Exploring these beliefs about the nature, cause or origin, duration, and consequences of the patient's health problem and the possibilities for recovery requires empathic listening. Decoding what the patient is trying to say is a central and sometimes difficult task here. By finishing the interview with a short summary, you make a smooth transition to the physical examination.

Gathering Information – Physical Examination

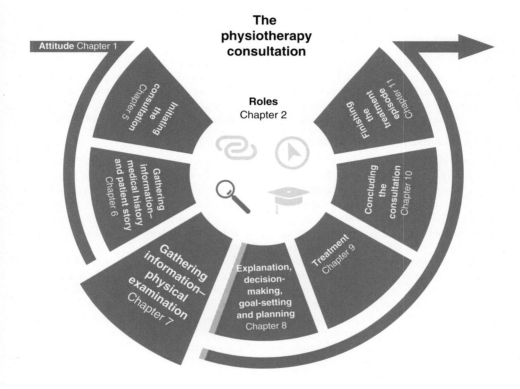

The physiotherapy consultation

Attitude Chapter 1

Initiating the consultation Chapter 5

Roles Chapter 2

Finishing the treatment episode Chapter 11

Gathering information– medical history and patient story Chapter 6

Concluding the consultation Chapter 10

Gathering information– physical examination Chapter 7

Explanation, decision-making, goal-setting and planning Chapter 8

Treatment Chapter 9

During the physical examination, which usually follows the interview during an initial consultation, you continue to gather information. This process consists of sharing information, obtaining more information, and establishing and explaining links. You continue communicating with the patient after taking their history in a similar way—you continue to work with them from the relationship of trust you have built up while analysing the health problem as a communicative detective, continuing to collaborate with the patient as much as possible.

Gathering information is often done by first sharing some information with the patient about the physical examination and then performing the test. In doing so, you try to include the patient as much as possible in your clinical reasoning process, without letting the patient feel that they are simply being examined as a passive object. During and after a test, you will try to obtain (additional) information by asking questions, among other things. As a follow-up to tests and assignments, you will regularly tell the patient what possible connections you have derived from the data obtained up to that point.

SHARING INFORMATION

During the physical examination and in the role of communicative detective, you try to help the patient participate in the process of analysing their own health problem in an appropriate and incremental manner. In your explanation, you pay attention to the fact *that* you want to investigate certain activities and functions, and you explain *why* you want to do a test and *what* it entails. The extent to which you share your explanation plays an important role in this: not too much and not too little.

Put Into Action: Sharing Information

Start the physical examination by briefly explaining that you want to examine various functions and activities that are related to the patient's complaints. You do this to involve the patient as much as possible in the physical examination. It is also good to let the patient know (again) that they are in control and that you are working with them by asking permission to start the examination. Say, for example, 'I want to have a look with you at how your ankle works. The investigation will not be limited to your ankle; we will also look at how your lower leg and knee function, because they work extensively in conjunction with each other. Is that okay?'

Sharing information during the physical examination consists of telling the patient why you want to investigate something. Then you explain the procedure (the execution of the test) and what you expect from the patient during or after the test. Sometimes it is more convenient to explain several tests all at once because they have broadly the same purpose—for example, a number of strength tests on a joint or a number of activities that are related to each other.

Sometimes it may be better not to explain the execution of the test in advance, but to do so during the course of the test itself. Say, for example, in the active straight leg raising test: 'I am now going to look at the strength and firmness of your lower back and pelvis (that is, the goal). Could you lie on your back with both your legs stretched out? (patient lies down) Good. Could you lift your right leg a tiny bit, stretched out (the execution)?'

■ Making Physical Contact

In (almost) every physical examination, you make physical contact with the patient. You touch them, test and examine the injured body part, palpate, move, etc. Touching and being touched is an accepted and acceptable part of a visit to a doctor or physiotherapist, including from the perspective of the patient. But physical contact always contains an intimate aspect. That's why it's good to ask the patient's permission before you touch them, on any part of the body. Say, for example, 'May I see how your wrist moves?' before you examine the patient's wrist. By asking permission, you show respect for the autonomy of the patient and awareness of the possible vulnerability of the patient in this situation.

In some cases, you consciously give no (or little) information in advance of performing a certain test. In these cases, you are interested in how the patient solves the movement/treatment problem in their own way. For example, you might say by way of introduction, 'I want to take a look at your running and jumping' and then give a specific assignment, such as, 'Could you walk across the street?' or 'Can you pick up this weight?' The information is thereby an instruction for the patient to perform an activity in order to achieve a specific goal (the 'what' of the movement). The way in which the patient performs the activity is up to them. That is why you omit the 'why' and the 'how' of the assignment in your instruction. Usually you use such an assignment for a specific movement to get an impression of the spontaneous execution of an activity. In cases like this, you make an exception to being communicative: you consciously give limited explanations, and let the patient figure out for themselves how to carry out the assignment.

It is important to keep the explanation of the purpose and execution of a test as short as possible. Give the patient just enough of an explanation to make it understandable to them and to be able to follow you in the reasoning process. It's best in this case to leave out the details, lest the patient feel overloaded with information. If you notice that the patient needs or wants more information, you can then give additional details.

Some of the things you want to test may be very complicated to explain to the patient. So simplify it! It's more important that the patient can continue to follow you than that they grasp and understand every single detail.

Explaining a test protocol is best done step by step, especially when the protocol is more extensive. You can then demonstrate what you mean by doing it yourself. If the protocol of the measuring instrument allows it, you can let the patient practice the procedure once, then start the test.

GATHERING INFORMATION

During the physical examination, you will obtain information by performing all kinds of tests. Conducting a test provides you with information. However, that information is not the only kind you can obtain during the examination. Throughout your physical examination, communication is an important tool for achieving an adequate outcome—for example, by asking questions, listening carefully, and observing non-verbal behaviour meticulously.

Put Into Action: Gathering Information

Both during and after a test, it is crucial to make observations. Of course, you already observe well enough to be able to determine the outcome of the test. But observing the non-verbal behaviour of the patient is just as important. Take a good look at their facial expressions, look for non-verbal behaviour in other parts of the body than the one tested, and watch how someone says something (intonation, volume, speed, etc.). The effort made or the degree of pain can regularly be 'read' better by looking at the patient's non-verbal behaviour than by what they themselves say about it.

To find out what the patient experiences during the test, you mainly ask open questions. After all, you want to know what the patient feels and notices. And in doing so, you want to influence the patient as little as possible. You should also regularly ask the patient more in-depth questions to probe their answers. By doing so, you can get more incisive answers from the patient about their experience during the test.

■ The Language of Therapists

With an important number of the tests you do as a physiotherapist, you want to know how the patient experiences the motion, whether they are in pain or not, and whether they feel or notice specific things. You ask them about these aspects, of course. But choose your moment to do so carefully: before, during or after the test. And think about how to ask the patient.

Pain Provocation Tests

Sometimes you want to gather information about very specific things, such as the presence of pain during a test. For a reliable answer, it is not wise to explain this to the patient when introducing the test. It is better to use wording that is more general, such as, 'I'm going to examine your neck movements now'. Appropriately directive questioning is also important. Do not ask the patient directly about pain, such as, 'Are you in pain?' By using the word 'pain', you are directing the patient unnecessarily; moreover, due to priming, they may also be inclined to refer to 'pain' too quickly. It is more reliable at such times to use less directive questions, as in, 'Would you mind telling me what this feels like?' or 'How is this for you?'

Muscle Strength Tests

When performing strength tests, the directive questions are often reversed. If you say you want to examine the patient's strength, they will probably be inclined to do their best. And that's exactly what you do want in this case. So say 'I want to examine how powerful your leg muscles are. Therefore, I would ask you to do your utmost during...'.

Other Tests

Words such as 'nerve' or 'joint' can often be sensitive or have a negative connotation for patients. Some patients have a bad association with having something wrong with their nerves or joints. The use of these words in your explanation of a test can thus cause alarm. Therefore, in neural tension tests such as the SLR (straight leg raise), it is probably wise to avoid the word 'nerve' and to use a more neutral formulation, such as, 'I'm about to lift your leg so that we can see how it goes'. You can also choose to say only what you are going to do ('lifting of the leg') without giving the purpose of the test.

In order to maintain good contact with the patient during a physical examination, you can pay attention to two things. First of all: listen actively to the patient by using (simple) reflections. Say, for example, if the patient does their utmost to make a move but fails due to a mobility disorder, 'I can see you're trying very hard, but it looks like you're not getting any further'. Try to keep eye contact where you can. Sometimes you can keep in touch by using a mirror, such as when you are standing behind the patient. This also helps the patient to see what you're doing. If you don't have to stand behind the patient, then don't.

As your physical examination progresses, it may be helpful to summarise the information you have collected up to that point. By doing so, you keep the patient involved, create a structure for them, and give yourself a good overview.

ESTABLISHING AND EXPLAINING LINKS

After performing various tests and assignments as a physiotherapist, you make all kinds of connections and come up with explanations. As a communicative detective, you don't keep this analysis to yourself: you involve the patient in the process. The frequency and depth with which you explain possible relationships and explanations to the patient depends on:

- the relevance of the information to the patient (and their process of analysis);
- the degree of firmness with which you draw a conclusion;
- the extent to which this information can affect the reliability of tests you still want to perform.

This is a tricky balance to strike. The tone in which you give the explanation to the patient should also fit these considerations; think of your choice of words and intonation.

Put Into Action: Establishing and Explaining Links

In the first instance, after performing a test, you give the patient feedback by telling them exactly what observation you have made. So, for example, you might say, 'You move less to the left than to the right', explain that 'The test shows that there is less muscle strength in the extensors of your knee', or note that 'This test seems painful for you'.

Then you can indicate the *meaning of* the finding from the test (or tests) in relation to the patient's complaints and their request for help. You then reason out loud about possible interpretations and analyses. For example, you might say, 'The reduction in muscle strength in your thigh means that you put unnecessary strain on your knee, which causes your pain while exercising' or 'Because you felt pain during these last three tests, I draw the conclusion that the pain in your shoulder has something to do with the tendons in your shoulder'.

In Consultation

Sharing information, asking permission, obtaining information	As we just discussed, I'm now going to examine your neck. Agreed? Would you mind pointing out to me again where you usually feel pain? *Usually here.*
Obtaining information (closed question)	And can you show me what movement increases the pain? *(turns their neck to the right and moves their head sideways, to the right)* Mmm, and can you also make that movement to the left? . . .
Obtaining information (open question)	How is it different? *Don't worry, this doesn't hurt!*
Obtaining information	And apart from the pain, what else do you notice? *I think I can move further to the left. When I move to the right, it also feels as if something is blocking the movement.*
Sharing information	Yes, you certainly don't move as far to the right. I would just like to feel the movement myself. So I'm going to hold your head and move your neck to the left and to the right. Try to relax as much as you can (test the movements to the right and left with a passive mobility test).
Making and explaining connections	Yes, that's obvious. The movement of your neck to the right is reduced and is also painful for you. So that confirms what I just told you—that your neck on the right side has temporarily less mobility, which is probably what is causing your neck pain. *Okay.*
Sharing information	All right. Now, I also want to look with you at the mobility of your shoulders and the part of the spine between your shoulder blades, because these areas in turn are important for the movement of your neck. Would you like to . . . . . .
Sharing information	In the meantime, I've been observing your posture. Something caught my attention. You have a strong tendency to hunch your shoulders and lean forward with your head (show what this looks like). Do you recognise that? *Yes, I try to stop myself doing it, but I'm often so busy that I forget all about it.*
Obtaining information (closed question)	Could you sit in the way you think you often sit? *(sits down with shoulders hunched and leaning forward, head in anteroposition) Something like that?*
Obtaining information	Mmm, this is what I've seen you do. Will you turn your head to the right? *(turns to the right, grimace of pain)*
Obtaining information	And to the left? *(turns to the left)*
Obtaining information (open question)	How's that for you? *Yes, this hurts even more than when I did it before, at the beginning. To the right, at least. It's okay to the left.* Could you sit up straight? Try stretching your lower back a little, yes, good. Now turn to the right and the left. How did that feel? *Yes, that's a huge difference! Turning to the right, I feel much less pain than when I sit hunched up. And it just feels smoother, easier. I can't believe it's that simple. But I'll never keep that up, sitting up straight all day!*

Continued

In Consultation—cont'd

Making and explaining connections	True, that will take some effort. I think that what we've just seen also plays a role in your health problems because you have a sedentary occupation and therefore probably sit in this position a lot. Can you suggest something you could do? *Yes, sure, I know I don't have a very good posture, no. Should I therefore always sit up straight?*
Making and explaining connections	Good question. Well, in any case, your posture puts your neck more often in a position where you will have less movement. If you want to turn your neck while hunched over, you're going to 'wring' your neck, so to speak. But if you sit up straight, it's much easier to turn; you've noticed that. If you stand, walk, and move, of course, this is even easier. You could say your neck is made to turn a lot. In some positions, this is easier than in others. And changing position as often as you can is possibly the best you can do. *Yes, sure.*
Summary/open question	So my message is actually this: make it nice and easy for your neck to move. How does that sound to you? ...

In Consultation

Sharing information	You have pain in your right groin and that's why I first want to take a look at the movements of your hip. I will also make comparisons with your left hip to determine what is normal for you. Would you like to lie down on your back on the table? *(lying down)*
Obtaining information *(neutral open question)*	Everything okay? Could you try to keep your leg as relaxed as possible, then I can feel it best. (lifts right leg) Just tell me what you're feeling. How's this? (makes an endorotation, looks at the patient) *Yes, I feel something now.*
Open question	Where do you feel it? *In my groin, where I always feel it.*
Open question	And what do you feel? *Slight pain.*
Neutral open question	And this movement, what is this like? (makes an exorotation, looks at the patient) *Ow! (grabs at their groin). Oh, yes, that's nasty. That's it.*
Reflecting	And in that exact place, by the looks of it? *Yes, yes.*

Summary

In this chapter, we have once again seen the communicative detective at work. Gathering information during the physical examination consists of three parts:

- sharing information;
- obtaining information;
- establishing and explaining links.

When sharing information, you briefly tell the patient that you want to investigate something, what it is, and why it is useful. In doing so, you are also talking about what you expect from the patient. By explicitly involving the patient in the analysis process, the assessment yields more. When gathering information, you mainly ask open and in-depth questions and pay attention to the patient's non-verbal expressions. Finally, by establishing connections between what you have found and explaining these to the patient, or by being communicative, you enable the patient to participate in the analysis process of the physical examination to the best of their ability. A particular focal point during the gathering of information is the language used by the therapist.

CHAPTER 8

Explanation, Shared Decision-Making, Goal-Setting and Planning

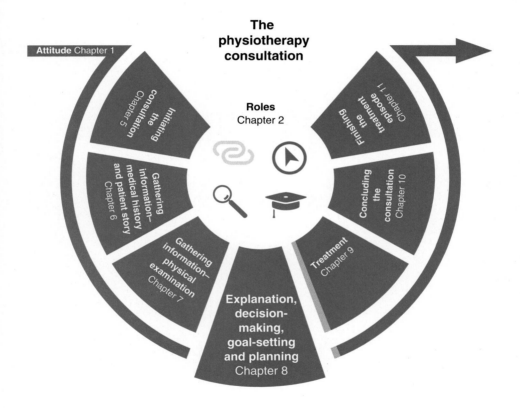

In the fifth core task of 'explanation, shared decision-making, goal-setting and planning', you and the patient choose the physiotherapy treatment together. In this process, you once again employ the role of a communicative detective.

The process of shared decision-making is done in eight steps (Epstein *et al.*, 2004; Kortleve, 2015; Scobbie *et al.*, 2013; Stevens *et al.*, 2017):

1. Present an analysis of the health problem.
2. Formulate the definitive request for help and the main goal.
3. Translate the main goal into sub-goals.
4. Prioritise sub-goals and offer choices.
5. Discuss the effort made, side effects, and pros and cons.
6. Negotiate and elicit values.
7. Check the patient's understanding of the problem and the options available.
8. Make choices.

In some situations, it makes sense to involve others in the decision-making process. When working with younger children, the parents naturally play an important role in the decision-making process. Informal carers and adult children are frequently involved with decisions regarding the elderly. Finally, it is possible for other care workers to participate in the decision-making process. The eight steps of the shared decision-making process are elaborated in below.

Once the choice of an approach has been made, the physiotherapist will formulate a plan with the patient and execute it. Here it is essential that the patient takes responsibility themselves. As a care worker, you play an important role in this through your communication approach: you must give sufficient space and time for the patient to take responsibility. A complication here is the 'ambivalence' that often plays a role in patients. Ambivalence means that the patient simultaneously sees advantages in the agreed approach and disadvantages with the result, leading them to take too little responsibility and no action. This situation will be discussed in the last section of this chapter.

PRESENT AN ANALYSIS OF THE HEALTH PROBLEM

During the previous core tasks, you 'included' the patient in your clinical reasoning process as much as was advisable. Now, much of the analysis of their health problem is known to them, at least in part. It's good to summarise this and make sure the patient understands you. It may be that certain things have eluded the patient, so you will have to check these points.

The physiotherapy analysis of a health problem is not the same as a medical diagnosis made by a doctor. The condition is usually not central to the physiotherapy analysis, but the consequences of the condition are, resulting in disorders or disabilities in activities and participation; the way the patient deals with the condition, whether consciously or subconsciously; the cause and the factors that have led to it; the factors that impede and promote recovery; and so on. This can make presenting your analysis and providing information about it complicated. At the same time, this is a crucial step. After all, to a large extent, patients behave on the basis of their perceptions of their health problem. With the information you offer, you want to influence the patient's perception of their health problem so that they are able to make a correct and informed choice about the treatment approach.

Presenting the analysis of a health problem is not one-sided; rather it is an interactive process. While presenting, you continuously check whether the patient is taking in and understanding your information. As you do this, you are already adjusting your approach: you adapt what you say and how you present it according to the patient. It may be useful to use a dialogue model such as the infographic discussed in Chapter 6 in the Section "Establishing and explaining links", especially in the case of complex health problems.

Put Into Action: Present an Analysis of the Health Problem

Presenting the patient with an analysis of their health problem takes place in three steps; you may recognise these steps from the Section "Sharing information" in Chapter 6 (prompt – share – prompt).

- **Step 1 - Prompt:** Find out what the patient already knows and ask permission to share the analysis of the health problem with the patient.

  First ascertain the patient's prior knowledge by asking a question. This 'activates' their brain. If you already have an idea of the patient's knowledge about the situation, first summarise it and check whether the patient may know more about it. In this summary, you immediately take into account things you have already explained (in the previous core tasks). Finally, ask the patient's permission to share the analysis of their health problem with them.

- **Step 2 - Share:** Explain the health problem.

  Connect to the patient's prior knowledge with new knowledge about their problem. When offering information, use the 'chunking method', which means that you provide the information in chunks. Explaining is like laying a brick wall—you need a good foundation (which is what the patient already knows) or to lay this foundation yourself (basic information). After that, you build the 'wall of information' brick by brick. While 'laying the bricks', you constantly check whether the patient understands you.

- **Step 3 - Prompt:** Ascertain if the patient understands the analysis and ask what this means for them.

  The last step stimulates the patient to better understand and then apply the information you have just provided. You also promote the acceptance of your message during this last step.

  With this in mind, first check whether the patient has understood, ask what else they want to know, and ask 'What do you think of this?' or 'If I tell you like this, what does this information mean to you?' Finally, in order to strengthen the acceptance of what you have said, you can ask 'Does this make sense to you?' or 'Are you convinced that this is the explanation of what's happening with you?'

Some points to remember when giving explanations include (Gaston & Mitchell, 2005; Houts et al., 2006; Kilkku et al., 2003; Shaw et al., 2009; Taylor, 2009):

- avoid jargon; use clear and simple language;
- use short sentences;
- at first, only give the essentials and be definite;
- enrich your information by using different 'communication channels': verbal, visual (images, film, diagrams, written information, etc.), imaginative (metaphors), self-experience/feeling;
- keep in mind that the patient can only remember a certain amount of information.

FORMULATE THE DEFINITIVE REQUEST FOR HELP AND THE MAIN GOAL

Following the analysis you have just presented, you consider the main goal which the patient has in mind for the physiotherapy treatment.

Often, the patient's main objectives are at the level of daily activities or participation. The opening question posed by the physiotherapist is important: it must lead the patient to thoroughly consider what they really want to achieve with the treatment. Good opening questions, depending on the patient and their health problem, could be: 'What would you like to do again but better?'; 'What would you really like to be able to do again?'; 'What can you hopefully do after treatment that you can't do now?'; 'In your opinion, when would the physiotherapy support be a success? what will you have achieved?'

Patients who experience a lot of pain symptoms may be inclined to set their main goal in terms of pain (i.e. at the level of disorders). This is, of course, logical, as pain severely impedes the patient, and that leads to them focusing mostly on this. Try to help the patient look at this goal in terms of activities or participation. Investigate which activity or form of participation they can no longer (or only partly) perform because of the pain and what they would like to change.

When formulating the objectives, the physiotherapist allows themselves to be guided in terms of content by the available evidence and by their own expertise. In doing so, they ensure that the ultimate goals are realistic and achievable. The most important conversation skills that the therapist uses are listening, reflecting, questioning in depth, and summarising. Try to listen to what the patient wants to say, and try to reflect to show that you understand them. You can also use in-depth questions to help them set the right goal and summarise what is said to create structure and clarity.

In the end, the physiotherapist usually presents the patient with a formulation of a therapy objective. Together, they improve this where necessary.

TRANSLATE THE MAIN GOAL INTO SUB-GOALS

In order to achieve the main goal, it is often necessary to set sub-goals. The patient must know these sub-goals and the relationship of each with the main goal must be clear to them. This will make them more motivated to work to achieve both the smaller steps and the larger goal. These sub-goals are often at the level of activities or functions. In your role as a communicative detective, you use your professional expertise to present and discuss the sub-goals with the patient.

PRIORITISE SUB-GOALS AND OFFER CHOICES

When the sub-goals are clear, try to prioritise them. Here, too, professional knowledge is essential to employ, in addition to the patient's personal preference. If, for example, resuming sports practice for 1.5 hours is the patient's main goal, then the sub-goals specify what needs to be done to achieve this overall aim. For example, you might first improve mobility and then improve muscle endurance to be able to complete simple, light workouts of 45 minutes.

Depending on the situation, the physiotherapist more or less takes the lead in this, taking the patient's preferences into account as much as possible. For example, in rehabilitation after cruciate ligament injury, the physiotherapist takes the lead in prioritising sub-goals. The steps in this rehabilitation are determined to a large extent by knowledge and insights from physiology and evidence-based rehabilitation. On the other hand, when improving activities of daily living (ADL) after a stroke, the patient needs to be in charge. After all, they can best decide which activities they consider most important and which they would most like to be able to carry out again.

The next step in the shared decision-making process is to offer choices regarding the treatment: How can you effectively achieve the sub-goals? You present choices based on the evidence available and your expertise. As far as possible, you indicate the chances of achieving the sub-goals for the various treatment options. In the physiotherapy treatment, the chances of a result are not always sufficiently known. You have to make an estimate for the individual case of the patient and communicate this to the patient in an appropriate way, not any firmer than is realistic. In order to keep an overview in mind, it may be helpful to write down the sub-goals and treatment options for the patient.

■ **Choices**

You can make or offer choices in physiotherapy on different levels. At the most fundamental level, you have to decide: physiotherapy treatment or not? Deciding not to have treatment often includes 'active surveillance'. In this case, we do not treat or intervene directly, but wait and see what the natural recovery brings. It is also good to inform your patient about this option, simply because it is effective in some cases.

If a physiotherapy treatment has been chosen, there is a second level at which decisions have to be made, namely: What is the goal (or main goal and sub-goals), how is the (sub)goal used effectively, and which method of working suits the patient?

DISCUSS THE EFFORT MADE, SIDE EFFECTS, PROS AND CONS

In this step, you discuss the amount of effort needed, side effects, and pros and cons of the different possibilities with the patient. Often, the amount of effort needed for different treatment options differs. Sometimes certain side effects are known to occur, although these are usually limited within the physiotherapy field. The various treatment options also have known advantages and disadvantages. Finally, there are advantages and disadvantages for the specific situation of the patient. In your role as communicative detective, you list all of these options and discuss them with the patient.

NEGOTIATE AND ELICIT VALUES

In this step, under the guidance of the physiotherapist, the patient examines what suits them best. What do they prefer and why? The physiotherapist guides the patient in weighing up the treatment options. What do they value most about their recovery? What are the strengths and weaknesses with regard to their own contribution? Do costs still play a role? Are adjustments to the approach possible and/or desirable so that they are better suited to the patient (e.g. are they easier to stick to)?

CHECK THE PATIENT'S UNDERSTANDING OF THE PROBLEM AND THE OPTIONS AVAILABLE

Before the physiotherapist makes the final choice with the patient, it is necessary to check whether the patient has understood everything so far. In order to check this, it is not enough to ask 'Have you understood?' because the patient will often give the answer which they think is socially acceptable. It is better to ask the patient if they can say it in their own words. Ask, for example, 'This information is complicated. I'd like to make sure I've explained it correctly. How would you sum up my story in your own words?'

MAKE CHOICES

In the end, the patient and the physiotherapist make a shared decision. Because they do this together, both the patient and the physiotherapist 'commit' to the decision.

■ **The Decision-Making Process**

The decision-making process, as elaborated here, describes all eight steps in detail. In daily practice, it will often be the case that the extensiveness and depth with which you apply a certain step will depend on the decision at hand. Some decisions are comprehensive and fundamental. An example of this is deciding whether or not a young man aged 19, with brain damage that occurred three years previously, should receive physiotherapy treatment in a rehabilitation centre. Other decisions are clearly less 'big' and fundamental, such as deciding how intensive the therapy should be in building up active stability of the ankle after a partial ligament tear in a young 25-year-old woman (i.e. doing a lot at home and having a consultation once every 10 days with the physiotherapist, or exercising two or three times a week under the guidance of the physiotherapist in their practice).

Depending on how comprehensive and fundamental the decision is, as a physiotherapist you also determine how long you take for the different steps in the process. Lastly, in daily practice, it is not unusual if some steps overlap with each other to some extent.

TAKING RESPONSIBILITY AND DEALING WITH AMBIVALENCE

Where possible, as a physiotherapist, you try to make the patient take responsibility for their health problem and make them take personal action. However, it is not guaranteed that the patient will take that responsibility. Even if the decisions regarding the treatment have been made together and goals have been sought and found which are supported by the patient, that patient might not take personal ownership of the issue. The extent to which people are willing and able to take responsibility for their own behaviour varies, sometimes from moment to moment. Fortunately, this can be influenced by guiding the patient in a professional way. Whether the patient takes responsibility and actually takes action depends on many factors. Some of these are related to the stable characteristics of a patient; other factors are less stable and therefore easier to influence.

The patient may not be inclined to take responsibility for their health problem. This may be because they have developed a passive pattern of interaction with their previous care workers. These care workers may have started to act as problem solvers, such that the patient did not have to do much themselves. As a result, the patient is passive in every new contact with a healthcare practitioner because they have become accustomed to being treated in this way. It is helpful to realise that the patient does not consciously choose their behaviour—it has become a learned (subconscious and automatic) reaction.

■ Language of the Patient

The words the patient uses can be meaningful when it comes to taking responsibility. You may recognise the following scenario: The patient talks about themselves but says 'one' instead of 'I'. For example: 'Yes, that's right, but one finds it hard to keep up with the exercises'. The patient means, of course, *I* find it hard to keep it up.

Why are they doing this? Probably because they realise that they should persevere, but they can't and this makes them feel dissatisfied with themselves. In order not to let their own sense of failure become too personal, the patient therefore uses the word 'one' instead of 'I'. It's good to be aware of this depersonalising tendency in your contact with patients.

A second explanation for a patient's reluctance to take responsibility can be found in your own communication. It's possible you've been more dominant in the conversation than you've realised. You may already have taken on too much of the solution by yourself. Either way, a pattern of communication has emerged that maintains the patient's passivity. In motivational interviewing, the 'repair reflex' of the care worker is referred to in this context. This term indicates that the care worker is so eager to help the patient that they take the situation out of the patient's hands, thinking for the patient and possibly even acting for the patient. The result is that the patient becomes passive.

A third explanation is 'reduced health literacy skills', the skills one needs to manage one's own health. Health literacy skills include those such as reading, language skills, analysis, combining things, and applying them to yourself. This is discussed in more detail in Chapter 14 in the Section "Reduced health literacy skills".

A fourth explanation may be the patient's ambivalence with regard to their choices, even if they made them themselves. Ambivalence, also called 'internal doubt', is evident in many people pursuing (or considering) a change. Think of changes such as doing exercises or following advice. Even though the patient has made a shared decision with you, it is not guaranteed that they will then take action. Many patients *want* to take action, but are hindered in doing so by some of their own thoughts and feelings which go against the decision. One consequence of this ambivalence may be that the patient does not take action in the end or that they only keep up the desired change for a short period of time. This is a common phenomenon, which is further discussed in Chapter 13 in the Section "Ambivalence".

Finally, it may be that the patient does not take responsibility because they do not yet envisage the approach sufficiently. It is not yet clear enough what they should do, even though the therapist already has a firm idea in mind.

Put Into Action: Taking Responsibility

Taking responsibility has everything to do with establishing an equal partnership between you and the patient. Involving the patient in the care process right from the start and not turning them into a passive object is therefore crucial. Once there is a good partnership and the patient is participating to the best of their ability in the care process, you simply need to continue this conversational style. Suppress the repair reflex ('I'll tell you the best thing to do') and use directive questions which activate the patient and reflect the patient's statements. Ask, 'How could you solve that' instead of explaining the solution (again). Or say, 'You've been exercising for a long time and very consistently as well. What helped you to do that?' Make sure you alternate your questions sufficiently with reflections to ensure that the patient feels understood and supported.

In addition to this approach, the following strategies are suitable:

- Use scaled questions by asking the patient 'Do you think you're going to be able to do this? Would you like to give a figure between 0 and 10 for this?'. Now the patient has to commit to whether they think they will succeed or not. If the score is low, you can then explore how the patient has arrived at this low mark and help them think about solutions to improve this.
- Use directive and solution-oriented questions. By using directive open questions in your conversation, focused on the solution, you get the patient to do some thinking. Furthermore, you more or less determine their 'mindset' because you are already being directive in your question. Ask, for example, 'What would make it better if you…', 'What could make it work for you this time?', or 'You mention a few things that make it difficult for you to work on this. What would make it easier for you?'
- Make things measurable with clinimetrics (e.g. performance tests) so that the patient can decide for themselves whether they are moving forward. After all, responsibility and self-management have a lot to do with patient involvement. Also, by using measurements that the patient can employ at home, such as an exercise app or 'activity tracker', you enable the patient to monitor their own behaviour.
- Make things clear to the patient, not just once, but repeatedly! Patients want to understand things; they look for logical connections. That is why people want to understand their health problem: so that they understand why certain forms of therapy are useful and others are not. But the knowledge required for this often slips away again and then the patient resorts to 'old' ideas and knowledge. That is a very good reason to regularly return to things you have explained before, for example by asking about them.

- Create an action plan to make a definitive transition from objective to behaviour. What exactly does the patient have to do, at what moment, how often, and how do they make sure they don't forget (e.g. what can be a reminder)? As a physiotherapist, you give input to this action plan by telling the patient, for example, which exercise they can do. Afterwards, the patient can decide where and when to do the exercise, how to make sure they don't forget, and that they exercise consistently. It is best to coach the patient by asking them to describe out loud what they will do, when, and how they will make sure they don't forget: 'Can you describe exactly what you're doing?' or 'Can you imagine what exactly it looks like?' In the end, you coach the patient in such a way that they formulate an action plan, with themselves as the subject. For example: *To make sure I exercise every day, I do two exercises every morning and every evening while brushing my teeth. The other two exercises I do every day after breakfast and after dinner. I will ask my wife to remind me and I will also stick a note in the kitchen next to the table so I won't forget to exercise after breakfast and dinner.*

- Write up a coping plan with the patient for those times when the patient expects it will be difficult for them to do what is needed. In practice, a coping plan is an emergency plan for difficult times, such as doing exercises when you don't feel like it at all. It is good to ask specifically about such times, especially when the patient has to do certain exercises for a long period of time or has to follow advice for the long term. Simply by thinking it through beforehand with the physiotherapist, patients may more readily overcome barriers and difficult times. The coping plan describes how to act or react in a certain difficult situation. For example: *If I don't feel like exercising, I imagine I'll get back pain again tomorrow. I then think about how annoying it is for me, how hard it is for me to handle it when I have backache, and all the things I can't do anymore.*

Finally, two points may also help ensure that the patient takes 'responsibility'.

First, it is important to ensure that your clinical reasoning skills and domain-specific expertise are at a sufficient level. What that level should be depends on the complexity of the patient's health problem. Therapists who don't have the required knowledge about a particular health problem will be unnecessarily ambivalent if a treatment doesn't seem to work. As a therapist, you have to exude confidence in yourself and your knowledge. This trust and energy lead to the patient being or becoming less hesitant or passive. So be careful not to feign knowledge with patients with a complex health problem. In such a case, contact a more experienced colleague.

Second, some advice: hang in there! Patients who have become passive have often become 'practised' in this type of behaviour. And so they are 'good' at it; a strong and persistent pattern has emerged in their behaviour. There's no blame to be had here; it simply is what it is. In these cases, it is best to persist in stimulating a sense of responsibility in the patient—otherwise, before you know it, you will be just another problem solver and the patient will undergo treatment without making an actual contribution. So hold on and break the pattern!

In Consultation

Request permission	Would you like me to set it all out for you? *Yes, please.*
Explanation/summary of health problem analysis	Like I just explained to you, you have a tennis elbow. I can imagine that's a pretty confusing term, since you don't play tennis at all. *Yes, that's right.*

Continued

In Consultation—cont'd

Sharing information	Well, a tennis elbow occurs in tennis players, but also in people who don't play tennis. It all has to do with the powerful squeezing action of your hand. In truth, it should be called a 'squeeze elbow'.
	Oh, in that way. Yes, as a carpenter, I do quite a lot of squeezing.
Open question (sharing information)	Exactly. What do you think a tennis elbow is?
	Um, yes, that's a good question. Some kind of an inflammation or something in your tendons?
Sharing information	Mmm, not quite. It is indeed in most cases a problem with the tendons of your elbow. Inflammation just isn't the right term.
	Oh, what is, then?
Sharing information	A tennis elbow is a painful irritation of the tendons of your wrist and hand at the level of your elbow. Look, here in this picture you see these tendons. There's no rupture, no inflammation, no damage. The strain creates an irritation that causes pain, comparable to muscle pain caused by vigorous exercise. This often makes the tendon temporarily stiffer and less flexible. The tricky thing about this is that it often causes you pain and you tend to spare your elbow as a result. This further reduces the flexibility of the tendon. And it often becomes a little more painful. Which makes you move a little less, and so on.
	Mmm, that's clear. Some kind of vicious cycle. It's logical.
Sharing information/ establishing links	Yes, that's right. So the job you did after that caused the pain in your elbow, mainly from squeezing with your hand. And you were doing this while holding your elbow almost completely straight, which placed your forearm muscles in an adverse position. As a result, there was clearly more elongation on the forearm tendons. This has most likely caused a strain, with the current painful irritation as a result.
	Yes, a concurrence of events.
Reflecting/controlling the concept of the patient	Yes, probably just a case of bad luck and not a weak spot or a vulnerability or something. What do you think of this so far?
	Well, it sounds logical and clear to me. I've just overloaded my elbow muscles and it's good to hear that there is no inflammation.
Formulating definitive request for help and main objective	Good. Now the question is: how do you get rid of your tennis elbow? Because that's why you came to me, right?
	Yes, exactly. I can't do my job properly at the moment, so I really want to get rid of it. Completely and, if possible, quickly!
Formulating a definitive main goal	Mmm, so getting back to work without being bothered by elbow pain would be the goal of the treatment?
	Yes, sure. Working without pain in my elbow is what I want.
Reflecting	You will then be satisfied with the result.
	Exactly.
Translating main goal into sub-goals	To achieve that goal, I think it is important that you get back the previous level of flexibility in your elbow and tendon, that you don't put too much stress on them again, and at the same time, keep moving enough.
	Mmm.
Open question	Putting too much or too little stress on your elbow is, of course, something that is mainly your responsibility. What do you think?
	Well, that could be tricky. I don't move too little, but maybe sometimes too much, because of my profession.

In Consultation—cont'd

Reflecting	It could be hard to avoid a lot of strain on your elbow in your line of work. *Yes, a little bit. I'd like to be clear about what I can and can't do.*
Sharing information	All right, I can help you with that. Let's come back to that later when we make things more definite. In addition, the flexibility of the tendon in your elbow plays a role. There are several ways to approach that. Would you like me to explain it to you? *Yes, please.*
Sharing information	Well, first of all, it is known that most tennis elbows are eventually resolved without treatment. But there needs to be a good balance between stress and rest, otherwise the tendons will not regain their flexibility. That takes six months to two years. *Okay.*
Offering options to choose from	The second option directly connects to this, namely that I will guide and coach you for a while to help to ensure that you indeed move sufficiently, don't suffer stress, and do not continue to avoid movements subconsciously. I expect that four consultations spread over three to four months will be sufficient. I will mainly coach you, give you exercises, and do them with you. *Mmmm.* The third option is that I offer you treatment three to four times every month with some specific techniques. This should bring back the flexibility in the tendons. Nature will do the rest; altogether, this will take another two to three months. *Mmmm.*
Discussing opportunities, effort, side effects, pros and cons	With each of these options, you have to take into account that when the pain decreases, you still have to temporarily avoid very intensive stress. It will still take some time for your tendons to fully recover. In all three options, I expect you to be able to continue working with some adjustment, although some movements will remain painful for a shorter or longer period of time. I don't think it's wise to make a lot of movements like the one which caused the problem. I estimate that all three options would have the same result. *Okay, so it's not necessarily essential to treat it, I can just wait and see?*
Discussing opportunities, effort, side effects, pros and cons	Yes, that's right. However, because you are avoiding certain movements now, you have to make sure that you completely and regularly stretch out and also bend your elbow. You probably have to make yourself aware of that every day, especially in the beginning. *Yes, that's true. Of course it's best to get started quickly.* Mmm. *What if you treat me in the next few weeks?* Option three, you mean? *Yes, exactly. How would that work? Is that painful?* Well, that can be painful. I'll do all kinds of elbow stretching in three or four treatments. And during stretching, it can hurt, and many people find it also hurts in the following few days. Especially after the first treatment, you often see some increase in pain. In the subsequent treatments, this almost always decreases.

Continued

In Consultation—cont'd

Negotiate and elicit values	*I see. I have to say I am leaning towards the second option.* Mmm, why is that your preference? *Well, I actually want to let nature do its work by waiting for the healing, but I do need a safeguard to make sure I stay aware of what I do and don't do with my elbow. And I want to make sure that I make the right movements to make everything flexible again. Especially with my work. I also feel that this is the best way to ensure that I can continue to do my job until I retire.*
Reflecting	You want to make sure you don't get this problem repeatedly. *Yes, I have to be careful with my body. Yes, I think we should do that.*
Check if the patient understands	Mmm. Just to be sure, before we make a decision, I'd like to make sure I've explained it to you properly. In your own words, could you summarise the three options? *Well, um, firstly, just to go ahead and let nature do the work by using my elbow properly. Secondly, the previous option but with your help to make sure I don't get sloppy. And the third is that you're going to give me a few treatments.* That's right. And what form does my support take if you go for option two? *Well, that I have an occasional consultation with you to keep me focused. So that I don't do too much, but also not too little, and bend and stretch my elbow enough to regain flexibility.*
Making a choice	Sure, a fine summary. You choose the second option, and we'll get started.

The following conversation fragment is an example of a conversation in which shared decision-making takes place and in which the physiotherapist subsequently works out an action plan and a coping plan with the patient. The patient suffers from Parkinson's disease.

In Consultation

Formulating a definitive main goal	Earlier in the conversation, you indicated that lately, you have been suffering increasingly from feeling stiff, especially when walking. And you would like to be less bothered by it than you are now. Is that right? *Yes, sure. Because of the stiffness and freezing, I am less independent at home and my wife doesn't want to leave me on my own. She's afraid something will happen to me. I find it pretty annoying myself, too. It didn't bother me as much in the past as it does now; it usually faded away. So it would be nice if with some exercises, I could deal with this better. Of course, I understand that this is part of my Parkinson's, but I have never had it this badly in the past and hope that it is still possible to reduce it by doing exercises. Especially while walking, it gives me problems.*
Summarising Questioning in depth (main goal)	I can imagine what a burden it is. And you said it correctly: it's part of your Parkinson's, but it's very well possible that I can teach you things that will help you deal with it better and make it easier for you. What would make you happy when it comes to walking? *Well, it really could be a lot better, but it does not have to be gone, I understand that I cannot expect that.*

In Consultation—cont'd

Translating main goal into sub-goals	Mmm, you are looking at this very realistically. Can I ask you to give me a percentage? How much of the freezing would you like to be able to solve on your own? *Well, if I manage to overcome it 50% of the time without anyone else's help, I'd be very happy. And as long as I don't fall or trip.*
Summarising	So your goal is to get yourself out of the situation half of the time when you stiffen up. And you don't want to trip when you get stiff. Is that right? *Yes, I think so. As long as it's feasible at least?*
Sharing information	For the most part, I think so. Reducing your fall risk to zero may not be possible, but a significant reduction is likely. *That's nice to hear.*
Offering options to choose from	My estimation is that we need about four weeks to achieve this goal, assuming that you regularly exercise and apply the things you learn. What do you think of that? *Well, I'll exercise for sure! I hope it can be done even faster.*
Discussing opportunities, effort, side effects, pros and cons	I can imagine. Experience shows that it takes some practice to master the solutions I will offer you. Only then can we get to the next step, which is to apply these techniques at the moment the stiffening occurs in your home or elsewhere. All in all, this takes at least four weeks. *Well, how are we going to do it?* Well, your motivation is great, that's obvious. Before we get started, I'd like to briefly discuss whether this is really the right choice for you. (After the patient definitively makes their choice, the physiotherapist explains, applies, and teaches the patient a number of techniques. Then the patient has to practice this at home.)
Creating an action plan (open question)	All right, we've now looked at three things you can apply when you freeze. I now want to discuss with you how you're going to practice and apply this at home. How often could you practice this at home? *Well, that's not an issue. I can practice this about five times a day or so?*
Creating an action plan	Mmm, five times a day could certainly pay off, so I think that's a good goal to aim for. Do you have specific times in mind for doing exercises? *Um, well, if I feel like it.*
Reflecting	You want to exercise five times a day and let this depend on whether you feel like it. *Mmm no, that sounds too casual. You're right. I'd like to get rid of this and so I have to make sure I actually exercise five times a day. If I do the exercises after every meal and after coffee or tea, then I'll get to five times.*
Creating a coping plan	Sure, good idea. That's something that has helped a lot of people. Does it make a difference whether you do it before or just after a meal and coffee or tea? *Oh yes, it might be better—to do it before, I mean. Then I exercise first and the food is my reward! Yes, that's a good plan.*
Creating a coping plan	What things could keep you from exercising? *Well, nothing I can think of.*
Request permission Open question	That's good to hear. May I explore this a little bit further? Have you ever had to exercise in the past? *Yes, sure.*

Continued

In Consultation—cont'd

Asking in-depth questions (open question)	When have you had trouble keeping it up? *Not at first. But once things were going well and I had fewer problems, I slacked off quickly.*
Making a coping plan	Yes, I understand. I hear that from other people, too. It's not an issue right now, but in a few weeks, we'll have to have a think about how to avoid this obstacle. What other things could keep you from exercising or have done so in the past? *Nothing comes to mind right now.*
Determining self-efficacy	Agreed. Now, if I were to ask: on a scale from 0 to 10, where 0 is 'no confidence at all' and 10 is 'I'm sure I can do it', what would be your answer? *Um, an 8.*
Reflecting	That sounds like a solid amount of confidence. *Yes, for sure!*

Summary

This chapter describes the climax of the diagnostic process: explaining the analysis of the health problem and arriving at shared decision-making. In the decision-making process, you set goals and make a plan together. This is a complex process in which the communicative detective is active.

Because it is not guaranteed that the patient will take responsibility for this shared approach, the role of coach has been further elaborated around this aspect. Through your style of communication and by making action plans and/or coping plans, you help the patient to take responsibility. Ambivalence in the patient can be a complicating element.

CHAPTER 9

Treatment

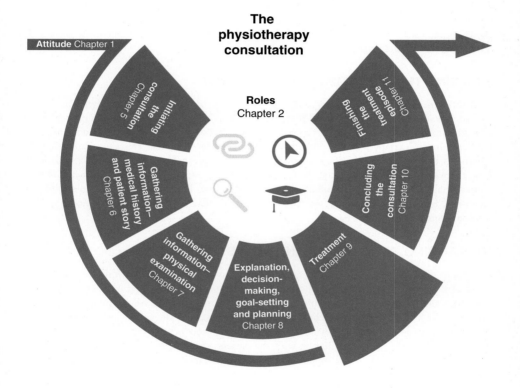

A physiotherapy treatment episode often consists of several consultations. In these consultations, which follow the diagnostic process, the implementation of the treatment plan and its evaluation is central. Your main roles are those of a teacher, coach, and communicative detective. Of course, the role of confidant remains important as the basis for all your communication.

A consultation during the therapy process starts naturally with greeting the patient, making contact, and looking back at the period that preceded the consultation. Subsequently, the physiotherapist and the patient look at the (sub)goals and evaluate them. Goals are then adjusted where necessary. Next, an intervention is initiated.

Physiotherapy treatment has various interventions. In a number of them, conversation plays a prominent role. This chapter will therefore also focus on giving instruction and advice to the patient. A step-by-step plan aimed at strengthening therapy compliance will also be discussed. Finally, we work out how best to provide advice. Because as a physiotherapist, you often want to influence the patient's behaviour and because this behaviour is partly based on the patient's thoughts and ideas, it is for your physiotherapy practice for you to be competent in providing advice in order to be able to influence these thoughts and ideas.

STARTING THE TREATMENT CONSULTATION

Every treatment consultation starts with a greeting. You have to focus your attention on the patient and the reason they are there. So make sure you don't start thinking about other things instead of focusing on your patient. You start the consultation in the role of confidant. Once the patient is in the therapy room, give them your full attention. A classic mistake is immediately looking at the patient's file on the computer. It's better to do this before you collect the patient from the waiting room. Use the first (half) minute in the therapy room to make contact with the patient, make them feel more familiar, and put them at ease. This has already been discussed in detail in Chapters 4 and 5. Then get to the point by reviewing the preceding period and the previous consultation.

MONITORING, EVALUATING, AND ADJUSTING GOALS

Consistent discussion of the physiotherapy (sub)goals is essential. After all, this is what it's all about. Are you and the patient still fully focused on these goals; is there progress, delay, or decline; what has caused this; is it in line with expectations; is it necessary to adjust the goals? In fact, these questions are all part of the clinical reasoning process that you follow as a therapist. It is important that you involve the patient sufficiently in this process in your role as communicative detective. By doing this in consultation with the patient, they remain involved and active. It is also easier to come to the shared conclusion that discontinuation of the treatment is the obvious course of action in the absence of a treatment result.

Put Into Action: Monitoring, Evaluating, and Adjusting Your Goals

When monitoring, evaluating, and adjusting goals, four focal points are important.

First of all, patients often forget things, including treatment goals. Regularly remind the patient of the goals they are working on with you. Not by giving a 'quiz' ('Why exactly does one do this exercise?') but by asking how the exercises are going and what they notice and reflecting on the answers. For example, 'How have the exercises gone in the last two weeks?' Next: 'You say it's going well; what makes you say that?' And then, reflecting the patient's answer: 'The exercises are getting easier and easier and you've noticed from your thigh muscles that you are starting to get stronger because you can hold on longer. That's good, because that's what we wanted to achieve with the exercises'.

You can also refresh the patient's memory by explaining the goal to them again. However, first ask the patient what they still know about the purpose of the exercises. Using a metaphor can be effective in your explanation. If you have used a metaphor with a patient before, you can often remind them of this effectively and quickly. Perhaps even asking for this metaphor may be enough to refresh the patient's memory. (In Section 'Giving advice', the use of metaphors is explained in more detail.)

As a second focal point: link measuring tools to the goals and make the results transparent for the patient. You may also wish to use a table or graph as a measuring tool so that the patient can track their progress. Simple performance tests are often very suitable for this purpose.

The third focal point is the patient's recollection of the situation before their treatment. Some patients forget what dysfunctions and/or disabilities they had before the treatment process started. This is especially true if this happened a while ago or if progress has been very gradual. The patient may then have the impression that nothing has been achieved, when in fact this is not the case. It is good to sometimes remind the patient of this by asking them about it or by naming actual disorders and/or disabilities, summing up the complaints, and giving scores from measuring tools so that a true picture is formed of the result achieved. It may also be desirable to name not only the rational issues, but also how the patient felt previously and how they feel now.

The fourth focal point concerns the possible lack of results. If the patient is familiar with the sub-goals of the treatment and knows what certain interventions are for (that is, which goal they are aimed at), it also becomes obvious to them if the treatment is having no effect. This insight is useful, allowing the patient to be more open to adjusting the therapy goals or accepting that the initiated treatment is not working.

GIVING INSTRUCTION

During many consultations, you will give instruction as a physiotherapist, partly in your role as a teacher and partly in your role as a coach. Instruction is about posture and movement, (movement) actions, and forms of movement. Clearly, this is a crucial part of physiotherapy.

When giving instructions about movement, it is important to realise that the patient is looking for logical connections in your instruction, such as between the instructed movement and the complaints they have. They may also look for the relationship between the exercise and the set goal. In other words: if you give instructions, you are also heavily involved with the patient's thoughts and their illness perceptions. A unique aspect of the profession of physiotherapist is that at moments like these, you can simultaneously influence both thoughts and actions, and also the interactions between them. And thoughts and actions can also strengthen each other. By explaining how something is done and then allowing it to be physically experienced (or vice versa), both the patient's thoughts and actions can change. This is often a more effective tool than just a verbal explanation.

To make advice and instruction on exercise and movement clear, three situations are presented below:

- Instructions for exercise and movement (in practice);
- Instructions for exercise and movement to do at home;
- Advice on everyday posture and movement.

Before you instruct the patient, you want them to be receptive to your advice and instructions. Therefore, first ask permission to instruct the patient by asking, for example, 'Is it all right if I take you through some exercises now?' After receiving the patient's consent, you start your instruction. An instruction follows the following basic steps:

- Explain *what* the patient has to do;
- Explain *why*;
- Explain and show the patient *how* to do it.

In the first step, you briefly state what the intention is. In the second step, you give the patient background information so that they understand what purpose the exercise serves and how the exercise helps to achieve the treatment goals. In the third step, you instruct the patient exactly on how to do it, now using much more detail than in the first step. In this step, you also show what the movement looks like.

You can, of course, deviate from this basic outline, depending on what form and goal you are pursuing.

Giving Instruction for Exercises and Movements (In Practice)

Movement instruction can be applied during the therapy process in the form of a movement assignment, a movement regulation, or a movement description. Targeted use of these presentations should lead to the patient doing exercises or adjusting posture(s) and movement(s) in their daily life. Your presentations determine the way you work during the instruction. If you use the movement regulation as a presentation, you give detailed instructions for the movement to be performed. All steps—what, why and how—apply. With the movement description, you also apply all the steps, but you are less detailed and prescriptive. This is especially visible in the third step, the 'how'. In the movement assignment, the 'how' disappears completely and the 'why' is brief. After all, this is about the patient's spontaneous movement.

It is important to keep your instruction as concise as possible. Don't talk about it too much—just tell the patient what they need to know to do the exercise properly.

Giving Instruction for Exercises and Movements to Do at Home

The steps just mentioned are, of course, also important with instructions to exercise and move around at home. What is more complicated in this case is that the patient must be able to remember everything and correct themselves if necessary. The following step-by-step plan will help you with this:

- Use the steps 'what', 'why', and 'how', depending on the presentation (assignment, regulation, description). Ask the patient to perform the exercise (or movement).
- Coach the patient on the execution: correct them by asking questions and name each correction in the form of focal points and tips (avoid negative feedback in your corrections).
- Also give instruction on the subsequent exercise(s), thereby coaching the patient on the execution.
- At the end, ask the patient to demonstrate all the exercises to you and to mention the focal points each time.
- Consider whether it is necessary to write down the exercises along with making drawings, taking photos, creating videos (for example with the patient's own smartphone), using eHealth, and so on. Always make a note of the individual focal points.

Giving Instruction on Everyday Posture and Movement

If you want to instruct the patient about their daily posture and movement and how to independently correct these, it is important to start from the way the patient always does something. In this case, an instruction will usually start with a movement assignment in which you look for spontaneous movement (or a posture). Then ask if the patient notices anything and use directive questions focused on the aspect you want to teach the patient. Ask, for example, 'Is this an active posture for you or more of a passive one?' or, to be less directive, 'What do you now notice about your posture?' This allows you to follow up on what the patient is accustomed to doing. Moreover, your subsequent message is more likely to be taken on board. In your subsequent steps, you adjust to the desired posture or movement by means of explanation and/or an example and finally by letting the patient do it themselves.

The following step-by-step plan will help you with this.

- Ask the patient how they normally assume a certain posture or make a movement.
- Coach the patient by questioning them on how they do it.
- Tell the patient how the posture or movement could be different (and better) and ask them to perform that version.
- Correct the execution and name the corrections in the form of focal points and tips (avoid corrective feedback).
- Give instructions for the next posture/movement(s) while also correcting them.
- At the end, ask the patient to demonstrate all postures and/or movements and to indicate the focal points each time.
- Consider whether it is necessary to write down the posture and/or movement, make drawings of it, take photos or videos, etc. Always make a note of the individual focal points.

PROVIDING EDUCATION

Patient education is an extensive theme, enough for a whole book in itself. This section briefly considers the most important principles of educating patients.

A patient's behaviour is partly based on their illness perceptions. The patient thinks (to themselves) about what is going on and what they should do about it. They try to imagine a logical conclusion to it all. They then make decisions and behave on the basis of this way of reasoning or their 'concepts'. A concept consists of a number of interrelated illness perceptions, such as in the following statement by a patient: 'A tennis elbow is caused by too much stress, in my case too much squeezing'. Another example is this statement: 'I don't think the tingling in my hand is caused by carpal tunnel syndrome like the neurologist said. It's coming from somewhere around my neck or shoulder, I think'. If you estimate that a patient's illness perceptions—the thoughts and feelings which incline a patient to behave in a certain way—are unrealistic and unfavourable to the prognosis, you have a reason to consider providing education.

There are several common unrealistic illness perceptions or 'misconceptions' in patients' thinking and reasoning. The list below describes an increasing complexity in the patient's unrealistic illness perceptions. As these misconceptions become more complex, your education provision will correspondingly become more extensive and/or more intensive. According to research in the field (Mosley & Butler, 2017), there are patient misconceptions:

- based on a single piece of missing knowledge;
- based on a concept (e.g. some coherent illness perceptions as in the following statement: 'I can't move my arm upwards very well; a lot of exercise solves that');
- based on multiple concepts (such as: 'Once I'm in so much pain, I have to loosen myself up, otherwise I keep having problems');
- based on a set of coherent unrealistic concepts or a paradigm (such as: 'I've got a bad back, so I've got chronic back pain, it'll never go away').

When providing education, you try to 'get a grip' on the patient's individual knowledge, reasoning, and concepts, to thereby influence the patient's behaviour (Engers *et al.*, 2008; Foster *et al.*, 2008; King *et al.*, 2018). You do this from the role of a teacher. Education can cover various topics, such as the patient's health problem, pain, stress, lifestyle, exercise habits, and more.

Effectively providing education is complex. After all, there are many factors that determine whether provision of education has the desired effect. Think of the message itself and, of course, of the messenger. And don't forget the social environment of the patient and the patient themselves. From this basis, we'll cover in more detail the aspects of education over which you have direct influence: the messenger and the message.

Put Into Action: Providing Education

Appropriate provision of education takes a structured approach. The greater the number of concepts that lead to behaviour which hinders recovery, the more extensive and complex the provision of education becomes. A single concept is often easier to influence than multiple concepts, let alone a paradigm. Which interventions are suitable depends on the complexity of the situation.

The following metaphor may help you imagine this. The thoughts and concepts of the patient form a coherent whole, comparable to a sandcastle (Mosley & Butler, 2017). Trying to influence a single concept is like changing a few grains of sand in the whole structure. Influencing several concepts is like changing part of one of the towers of the sandcastle. Influencing a paradigm is like completely rebuilding one of the towers of the sandcastle. It follows from this that the larger the 'intervention' you want to perform, the more strategic your approach should be. 'More strategic' in this context means that the system (such as the structure) and the form of education provision become even more important.

The form of education provision depends on the degree of a particular patient's misconceptions. In the case of a minor misconception or a single concept, you are probably initially inclined to opt for a factual explanation, i.e. explicit knowledge transfer. You can also use concrete examples that are close to the patient's situation. When you want to explain more concepts, and the connection between different concepts and change through education provision, you need to make more use of implicit explanations. This means that you use metaphors and 'frames' to provide insight into the complex information and connections, without needing to explain all the knowledge in detail. You also allow certain concepts to be experienced personally or become evident from the patient's behaviour. By letting the patient reflect on this experience, you link the (learned) experience to the imparted knowledge and vice versa. This has been worked out in more detail in Figure 9.1. This diagram is meant as a rule of thumb.

Two focal points apply to any form of education provision.

First, make sure your explanation is always understandable and memorable. In other words, make sure your explanation is *so* understandable and memorable that the patient can explain it to someone else at a noisy birthday party. Strive to make your explanation 'birthday party proof'.

Second, before you can provide education or teach the patient, you want to prepare them by helping them to be receptive to what you want to explain. You do this by asking your patient's

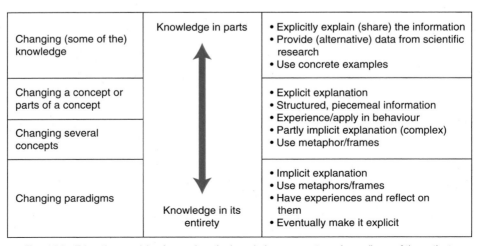

	Knowledge in parts ↑ ↓ Knowledge in its entirety	
Changing (some of the) knowledge		• Explicitly explain (share) the information • Provide (alternative) data from scientific research • Use concrete examples
Changing a concept or parts of a concept		• Explicit explanation • Structured, piecemeal information • Experience/apply in behaviour
Changing several concepts		• Partly implicit explanation (complex) • Use metaphor/frames
Changing paradigms		• Implicit explanation • Use metaphors/frames • Have experiences and reflect on them • Eventually make it explicit

Figure 9.1 Education provision focused on the knowledge, concepts and paradigms of the patient.

permission. After they give their permission, you start working together. If your education provision will be more extensive, make sure that the patient remains involved.

Next, we'll go into more detail to make the explicit and implicit approaches to learning more concrete. First, we'll examine the explicit approach and then the implicit approach.

The Explicit Approach in Education Provision
Education provision can take place by giving verbal (professional) information to the patient. The amount of information should be carefully paced. The consistency of the story as a whole is also very important. This means that it is necessary to think very carefully about what information you want to give, how you want to structure it, and how much time you want to spend on it. The more complex and extensive the information is, the more important it becomes to create an easy-to-follow story. Create 'chapters' in your knowledge transfer and make a summary at the end of each chapter. Make sure there is a connection between the 'chapters' by using connecting sentences.

When providing information, a number of points may be helpful:
- Support your story through the use of diagrams, drawings, images, and videos (Gaston & Mitchell, 2005; Houts *et al.*, 2006);
- Use jargon if it has a function, but never very often;
- Give the patient written material that supports the information you have given;
- Use online information that suits your story; for example, send it to the patient by email;
- Realise that your non-verbal communication is decisive for whether the patient ultimately accepts the message;
- Help the patient keep an overview in mind.

Chapter 15 discusses the reversal of unrealistic illness perceptions in patients with (chronic) pain.

The Implicit Approach in Education Provision
A metaphor is a form of imagery based on an equation. It achieves its effect through the associations it evokes. By saying that 'working on your recovery is like doing an elite sport', you automatically create the idea that recovery means strenuous exercise, without saying this explicitly. Moreover, 'an elite sport' has a positive connotation, which 'strenuous exercise' may not have. On the other hand, saying 'working on your recovery is a slog' would also give the impression that you have to work hard to recover, but in a much more negative tone.

'Framing' is a communication technique often used in political debates and in advertising. Using a certain frame (or image) conjures up a number of desired meanings more or less 'automatically'. The beauty of this technique is that you don't have to make these meanings explicit—but they will still enter the patient's mind. An effective frame can consist of just a single word. For example, the word 'warmth' has a positive connotation for many people with neck problems.

When using metaphors and framing, you implicitly teach the patient a new meaning which reveals a 'new' concept to them. The metaphor or frame is automatically accompanied by some meanings which you find useful, while not having to name them directly. You also do not bring in explicit knowledge that would lead you to describe the existing concept as incorrect. Instead, you use a metaphor or frame to make complicated things manageable and to subconsciously weaken strong concepts and gradually replace them with new, more beneficial ones. By connecting metaphors and frames to the patient's experience, the effect is further enhanced and the patient remembers the information better.

Several metaphors have been developed and made available on Evolve to give you ideas of how to use this tool. Here's one example to illustrate. It's about the role that exercise has for the health of our musculoskeletal system: 'Moving is like brushing your teeth. You have to do this every day to maintain your teeth properly. If you skip brushing your teeth too often, problems arise and the dentist has to set to work on solving them. You brush your teeth daily as a small bit of preventive maintenance. And as major maintenance, you have to floss a few times a week. Flossing for your dental health is like an hour's exercise a few times a week for the musculoskeletal system'.

In Consultation

Attunement Sharing information Asking permission	We talked earlier about the osteoarthritis in your knee. Then I indicated that exercising your thigh muscles could most likely reduce your pain and other problems. I want to talk to you about that so that you understand what we're going to do with the treatment, all right? What do you know about osteoarthritis? *Well, that's wear and tear! That you have less cartilage in your joint, right?*
Reflecting Sharing information (explicit learning)	Mmm, indeed, with osteoarthritis, the cartilage often becomes thinner. As a result, the ligaments of your knee joint will become slightly slack. Does that make sense to you? *Well, I can't quite understand that.*
Sharing information	Maybe the next model will help you? (explains with knee model) *That makes it a lot clearer. What about the pain? Is that because of the thin cartilage?*
Sharing information	Well, most of your pain is caused by the space in your joint due to the weaker ligaments, rather than the osteoarthritis of your knee and the thinner cartilage. *Okay, that's good to hear!*
Asking to apply something	By exercising your thigh muscles now and making them stronger, they more or less take over the function of the ligaments of your knee joint and the movement of your knee can become more robust again. As a result, your pain and other symptoms may gradually diminish. What do you think of this explanation? *Well, it makes sense. But I did have the idea that the pain was caused by the thin cartilage... but you've explained that already...* *Yes, so that's going to mean exercising!*
Sharing information Metaphor	Mmm. Exercising often helps with complaints like yours. An additional effect of exercising is that you move a bit more, of course. Well, that's actually a good thing! Exercise is necessary to lubricate your joint and the tissues within, thereby providing nutrition. Just like oil in a car engine. Regularly running the engine makes the oil circulate, which keeps it in good condition. *Yes, I've heard of that.*
Asking to apply something	Maybe you have felt this when you've been sitting down for a while and need to get going again?

Providing Education: Words You Should Not Use

While explaining something, your choice of words is crucial, especially when using metaphors and examples. Words differ in meaning and tone, and you want to strike the right chord when providing education: you want to convey the exact meaning that fits your explanation and the purpose of your explanation. The latter is especially something that you should keep an eye on: What is the purpose of your explanation?

Let's look at an example to clarify this. Here are a few statements which could be used to articulate a particular back problem:

1. Your back feels like it is stuck;
2. You have difficulty bending your back;
3. You find it hard to bend over;
4. You feel stiff in your back when you bend over;
5. Your back is limited in its mobility.

With all five of these statements, you could explain to the patient the reduced mobility of their back, but different words are used each time: *stuck, difficulty, hard, stiff, limited*. You may also notice that the verb changes each time and that what the verb refers to is not always the same.

This changes the meaning and sound of the statement each time: *feels like, you have, you find, feels, is*. In the first sentence, the person's *back* feels like it stuck; in the second sentence, the *person* has difficulty bending their back. The advantage of statements 2, 3, and 4 is that you are addressing the person directly, in contrast to statements 1 and 5, where you refer to the patient's back more as an object. The latter approach may also lead to the patient distancing themselves from their health problem and adopting a passive attitude.

Another aspect of language use is the use of personal pronouns. It is often better to say '*your* back' than '*the* back' if you mean the patient's back. Likewise, use '*your* leg' and not '*the* leg'. The reason for this is again the 'ownership' of the health problem. Formulations such as 'the back' and 'the leg' create distance between the patient and the injured part of the body, and the patient may not feel responsible for their health problem as a result.

Finally, words always have a certain connotation. Think carefully about what this is or could be in the patient's mind, and choose words that fit what you want to convey. Some examples of words with different connotations:

- problem/challenge;
- overload/overuse/strain;
- bad knees/vulnerable knees/sensitive knees;
- a limp/a less powerful gait;
- stuck/stiff/moving is less easy;
- unstable/wobbly/too movable.

Choose your words carefully. Think about what they mean and what you want to achieve with your explanation. A rule of thumb here is to make sure that the words you use can provide a positive perspective as much as possible while also taking the patient seriously.

Practicing New Concepts

A unique aspect of physiotherapy is that much of what you explain to patients or teach them can be experienced or practiced together with the patient. After giving some explanation or deploying a metaphor, you can try out the concept directly with the patient in an exercise or movement and let them reflect on what they feel and think when they do this. If you have a patient with a torn ankle ligament, for instance, you can explain to them that using their ankle in a certain way will not overload it (such as putting stress on the ankle while in a neutral position). You can also apply this immediately. Invite the patient to use their ankle as you explained earlier. Also ask the patient what they feel and what they think. So if they feel pain, ask them what they think about it. Then ask what they think this means for their ankle (bad/not bad?/can it hurt?).

By using this strategy, you are more likely to get the patient to understand the new concept properly. Moreover, you create a learning cycle (Figure 9.2).

GIVING ADVICE

In addition to instruction, you also provide the necessary advice to the patient. This advice comes out of analysing the health problem and the goals you have set together with the patient. Advice can be given on matters such as the extent to which and the way in which the patient puts strain on their body, their lifestyle, their work–life balance, the desired amount of daily exercise, daily movements, and any 'tricks' involved, etc. Advice that the patient consistently follows can contribute just as much—and possibly more—to their recovery than an exercise, mobilisation technique, or massage (Maher *et al.*, 2017; Malliaras *et al.*, 2015; Pauwels *et al.*, 2001).

Advice is linked to knowledge and motivation, which is why you are active in the role of teacher and coach when giving advice. You provide knowledge, link a piece of advice to it, and coach the patient in determining the value of your advice for their health problem.

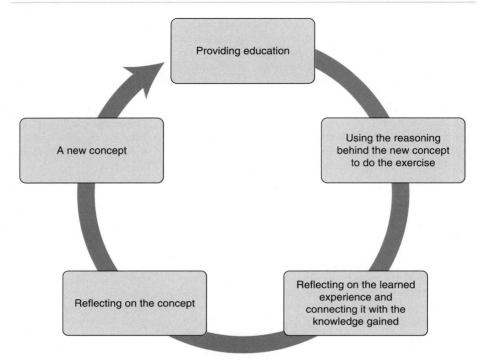

Figure 9.2   The learning cycle focuses on adjusting the patient's misconceptions.

Put Into Action: Giving Advice

Giving advice starts with asking permission to discuss your giving of advice. You then examine the patient's knowledge of the advice you want to give and provide additional knowledge. In Section 'Providing education', we already discussed the provision of education to increase knowledge.

In a step-by-step plan:

1. Ask permission to give advice. Say, for example, 'I'd like to discuss with you some advice that I think is important for your recovery; is that okay with you?'
2. Investigate prior knowledge by saying, for example: 'I'd like to talk to you about the extent to which you put stress on your knee. What daily activities are good to do, in your opinion?'
3. Provide additional knowledge by explaining to the patient those issues that have not yet been addressed.
4. Check whether the patient understands the information by, for example, asking them to summarise in their own words what you have discussed.
5. Now give the patient advice or ask what the patient thinks the information just discussed means for their situation, so that the patient formulates the advice themselves.
6. Come up with a specific plan to implement the resolutions. For this, you could ask: 'If we put this into action now, what do you plan to do yourself?'

PATIENT COMPLIANCE

Every healthcare professional knows that patient compliance is generally poor. It is striking that many care workers also seem to think that this does not apply to the patients they treat themselves.

The reality is probably that every physiotherapist has to take the figures of therapy compliance into account: at best, we can likely expect 50% therapy compliance, although 35% may be a more realistic percentage (Bassett, 2003; Wahl *et al.*, 2005). This is a good reason to make this a serious focal point as a physiotherapist.

Patients (and therapists!) make an implicit trade-off between 'What does it cost me?' and 'What does it get me?' This cost–benefit analysis results in ambivalence, and ideally the benefits should tip the balance to achieve patient compliance. This makes it clear how important it is that the physiotherapy targets fit in well with what the patient wants to achieve with their health problem, and that they have optimal insight into the connections between the interventions and the objectives.

The phrase 'therapy compliance' is actually a somewhat strange term to use in this book. The term implicitly gives the impression that the patient *follows* or *should* follow the instructions, education provision, and advice of the clinician. However, in patient-centred care, which is the starting point of this book, the patient is in control and the physiotherapist explicitly tries to pursue the patient's goals (chosen by the patient!) and tries to make a decision about the treatment together with the patient. The patient is not loyal to the therapy (or its 'prescriber'), but loyal to their own wishes. For the sake of convenience, however, we will use the term 'therapy compliance', because it is so commonly used in relevant literature and research.

Here are a number of suggestions for investigating and promoting compliance in daily practice.

Put Into Action: Patient Compliance

The starting point for strengthening therapy compliance is to have involved the patient in the decision-making process about their treatment and in setting goals. Yet this is no guarantee. What more can you do to promote therapy compliance?

First of all, you need insight into the extent of the patient's therapy compliance. In order to investigate this, the following steps, carried out from your role as coach, may provide some guidance:

1. Ask about therapy compliance. Watch your directive questioning; questions should be neutral, such as, 'How are the exercises going?' Also ask for specific examples, such as, 'How many times did you practice last week?' Avoid asking a closed question such as, 'Are you doing your exercises?' Listen carefully and think about what the patient says. If you are still in doubt about whether the patient's therapy compliance is sufficient, proceed to the next step.

2. Ask the patient to demonstrate the exercise and give a logical reason for the request—for example: 'Could you show me the exercises so we can make sure you're doing them correctly?' If the patient has already done the exercises many times, they are normally able to demonstrate them without help. Execution errors can, of course, occur, and you can correct these immediately. It's also important to take into account potentially reduced health literacy skills due to compromised health (see Section "Taking responsibility and dealing with ambivalence" in Chapter 8). If you still have doubts about the patient's therapy compliance, move to step 3.

3. Discuss your doubts. You can describe specific behaviour that you have observed, give your interpretation of it, and ask the patient for a response. In giving feedback to the patient, use an appropriate method. For example, you might say, 'I notice that you have an ambivalent reaction to my questions about exercising at home. I get the feeling you didn't do the exercises very often. How do you feel about that?'

In order to support the patient in their therapy compliance, it is important to regularly investigate and discuss this with the patient. Do this for at least the first three consultations, as for some people it can be particularly difficult to get going. Others have difficulty persevering, so with them it becomes more important to have these checks as time passes.

Strengthening Therapy Compliance

Should it turn out that the patient's therapy compliance is insufficient and the patient is aware of this, then you and the patient can investigate the cause together. Together with the patient, decide to discuss this topic to see what you can do about it. Next, you can explore, among other things, any of the patient's views that may be important in affecting their behaviour and compliance. Just like you do when exploring therapy compliance, you work on strengthening it from your role as coach. The following 'steps' (Bijma, 2012) may give you some guidance here. Feel free to deviate from this plan if you need to.

1. Discuss with the patient whether they feel it makes sense to take a closer look at their therapy compliance.
2. Examine who's responsible for what. What part of working on recovery does the patient see as their responsibility? Are they willing to take this responsibility as well?
3. What does the patient think about the usefulness of the exercises? Investigate the patient's beliefs in this area.
4. Investigate the patient's self-efficacy. How much confidence does the patient have in the correct way (execution/number/frequency) of doing the exercises and/or advice? Use a scale from 0 to 10 to help the patient grade their confidence, where 0 stands for 'no trust' and 10 for 'I'm sure it will work'.
5. What skills does the patient need and have? Skills involved in these cases are execution and motivation skills. Examples of execution skills include: the correct execution of the exercises, the ability to keep it up long enough, building up the number of exercises independently, and correcting oneself in the execution. Motivation skills include aspects such as planning the exercises, motivating yourself at times when you don't feel like doing something, fitting the exercises into everyday life, and setting and evaluating goals.
6. Does the patient experience obstacles? Discuss these and find solutions together.
7. Make an action plan. Action plans define what the patient is going to do and when they are going to do it. This helps the patient to translate their intention and goal into concrete actions. In Section "Taking responsibility and dealing with ambivalence" in Chapter 8, we briefly discussed how to draw up an action plan.

With each step, you engage from your role as coach. Apart from applying the above questions when you have doubts about the patient's therapy compliance, you can also use them immediately after you have assigned the home exercises.

Dealing With Ambivalence in Relation to Therapy Compliance

A common reason that patients don't do exercises or follow advice is that they are ambivalent. This phenomenon was already explained in Section "Taking responsibility and dealing with ambivalence" in Chapter 8. Because the patient is in conflict with themselves, and because the motivations in favour of the change ('exercising') seem insufficient in comparison to those against the change, the patient does not take action. Exploring the patient's ambivalence is very useful both because it gives the patient insight and because it gives you opportunities to coach them on this aspect. During this exploration, you can then see if you can let the patient elaborate on the motivations and aspects that argue in favour of the advice or exercises to be followed. This is further elaborated in Section "Ambivalence" in Chapter 13.

Summary

In this chapter, various aspects of communication during the treatment are discussed. The dominant roles here are the teacher and the coach.

Each and every consultation in the therapy process starts with you in your role as confidant: making contact and paying attention to the patient. In addition, as a communicative detective, you pay attention to how the patient is doing and how they feel with regard to the goals set. Your goals can also possibly be adjusted in consultation.

Providing instruction, in the role of a teacher, requires a well-considered approach. Depending on the presentation, your instruction will be more or less extensive: from very concise for a movement assignment to very detailed for a movement regulation.

In your role as a teacher, you also provide education to the patient. By working methodically, the effectiveness of the education provision increases. The extent and form of the education provision depends on the degree of the patient's misconceptions: from explicit knowledge transfer in the case of minor misconceptions to implicit forms such as metaphors and frames in the case of major misconceptions. Finally, it is very effective to share what has been discussed during the process of education provision with the patient.

Advising is a task of the teacher and the coach. You provide knowledge and help the patient to gain insight, after which you coach the patient further in applying this knowledge to themselves and their situation.

A particular focal point is the patient's therapy compliance. By systematically paying attention to this from your role as coach, you help the patient do what is necessary for their recovery. Self-efficacy and ambivalence are important aspects here.

CHAPTER 10

Concluding the Consultation

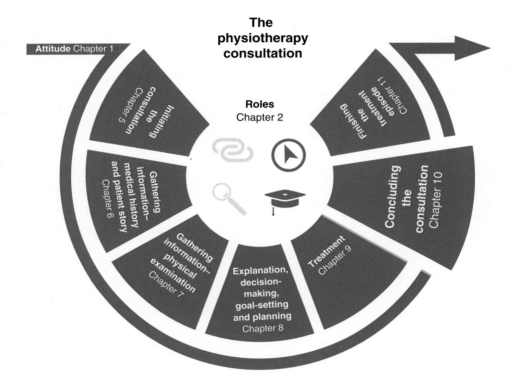

After all kinds of interventions have been carried out during the consultation, the time for the consultation is almost up. At this moment, it would be a pity to simply make a quick follow-up appointment and say goodbye to each other. If you conclude the consultation in a good way, you can improve the patient's involvement and ensure that the time until the next consultation is used optimally.

THREE QUESTIONS AT THE END OF THE CONSULTATION

At the end of the consultation, you will go through a brief summary of what you have done with the patient, the advice and agreements you have made, and how the treatment process will proceed. Three questions will guide your conversation with the patient:

- What will the patient do in the period until the next consultation?
- How will we proceed next time? Which goals are central?
- What will the physiotherapist do in the period until the next consultation?

The first and second questions support, among other things, the patient's self-management and therapy compliance. The third question emphasises working together: in the context of further treatment for the patient, the physiotherapist may have to find out things or arrange for certain items that are necessary for further treatment.

What Will the Patient Do in the Period Until the Next Consultation?

At the end of the consultation, in order to promote therapy compliance, you consider together what the patient is going to do in the time until the next consultation. This may include a summary of actions and exercises. Along with the patient, you can also name the goal you are working towards and tell them why a certain action is needed. And, of course, you also pay attention to the actual actions. You do this from your role as coach. Most effective is to let the patient take the lead in this summary by asking them, for example: 'We've been going through a number of exercises. To make sure I've explained everything correctly, I'd like to ask you to explain it to me. Would you like to do that?' And then after that: 'Good. We've also discovered that it's important to change the way you sit behind your desk. Could you sum up what you're going to watch out for and when you're going to do this?'

You may also wish to suggest that the patient writes things down as an *aide memoire* and a helpful reference.

How Will We Proceed Next Time? Which Goals Are Central?

A brief preview of the 'highlights' of the treatment process can support the patient by giving them an idea of what they are working towards. Say, for example: 'What we're working towards together is that within three weeks, you'll be able to work, and in five to six weeks, you'll be able to do a workout again'.

What Will the Physiotherapist Do in the Period Until the Next Consultation?

In concluding the consultation, the actions you will take in the interest of the patient should not be neglected. You may have agreed to find something, or to contact a colleague or arrange a referral. Mention those actions here, too. And put them in your diary immediately so you don't forget them.

Summary

In this chapter, we briefly consider concluding a consultation during the therapeutic process, based on the following three questions:

- What will the patient do in the period until the next consultation?
- How will we proceed next time? Which goals are central?
- What will the physiotherapist do in the period until the next consultation?

Finishing the Treatment Episode

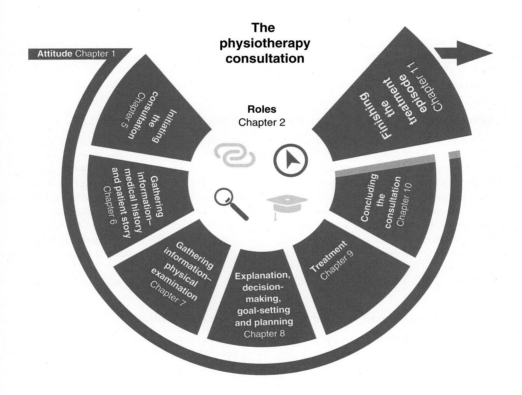

The physiotherapy consultation

Attitude Chapter 1

Initiating the consultation Chapter 5

Gathering information– medical history and patient story Chapter 6

Gathering information– physical examination Chapter 7

Roles Chapter 2

Explanation, decision-making, goal-setting and planning Chapter 8

Treatment Chapter 9

Concluding the consultation Chapter 10

Finishing the treatment episode Chapter 11

Ultimately, every treatment episode ends. In many instances, this is because there is a sufficient result or (almost) complete recovery and because the patient and you are in agreement. But that's not always the case. That is why, in this last chapter of Part III, we examine three ways in which you might conclude a treatment process. These are:

- The patient and you want to conclude the treatment process;
- The patient wants to conclude the treatment process and you don't (yet);
- You want to conclude the treatment process and the patient doesn't (yet).

There are various reasons or motives for concluding a treatment programme; for example, the treatment goals may have been achieved, partly achieved, or (almost) not achieved. Complications or a deviant course can also be reasons to stop. Finally, you may want to end the treatment process because of a disturbed or flawed relationship.

The three situations, described in combination with the reason or cause for concluding the treatment process, determine the complexity of the conversation that follows. The following sections give more detail on the three situations mentioned above, combined with the most common and most difficult reasons/causes. The role that the physiotherapist plays here is that of coach and possibly also that of communicative detective.

THE PATIENT AND YOU WANT TO CONCLUDE THE TREATMENT PROCESS

The most common situation is probably when the patient and you want to end the treatment process because the goals have been achieved in part or in full. In this situation, you operate in the role of communicative detective and coach.

At the end of the treatment process, there are all kinds of issues that may require attention. You evaluate the result; you may pay attention to continuing to work independently on therapy goals; and, if desired and applicable, you consider how to prevent recurrence. Finally, especially in the case of long-term treatment, it can be useful to evaluate the collaboration with your patient. Which aspects you perform extensively or just in a limited way (or possibly don't perform at all) are up to you.

Evaluation of the Result

Along with the patient, look at what you've accomplished. You are now active in the role of communicative detective. What's the patient's condition now and what was it at the beginning? It's good practice to use the measuring tools you have used before, as they are familiar to the patient. Recall the goal of the treatment and ask the patient whether they think it has been achieved or not.

If the treatment process is concluded because the treatment result is limited or absent, or if complications have occurred, you discuss with the patient the (possible) cause(s) and what you can learn from them. You also evaluate your contribution and that of the patient in order to obtain as complete a picture as possible.

Continue Working On Goals at Home

It often happens that the collaborative treatment process may conclude, but the patient continues to work independently on certain goals because not all their targets have been fully achieved yet. It is important to discuss these goals explicitly during the completion of the treatment process. Coach the patient in this and stimulate them to think about it themselves by asking them questions and letting them name the goals out loud.

It can be helpful to draw up an action plan together for a specific purpose. An action plan contains a complete description of movements in the first person so that the patient can relate to the activities immediately. The plan should preferably also be formulated by the patient themselves. An example of such an action plan is: 'I practice early every weekday morning just after I get up. I do all five exercises for my shoulder. I ask my girlfriend to support me for three months by reminding me when I am likely to forget. I also put a reminder in my diary'.

Emphasise that the goals and actions are important for the bigger picture. It's not about continuing to do an exercise 'because the physio wants me to'. It is all about carrying on doing a certain exercise for a purpose—for example, to prevent the patient from injuring themselves again or to be able to resume in the future those activities which they have been unable to do. And that could be worth a lot to the patient!

Even more than usual, it is now important to look with the patient at integrating the exercises into their activities of daily living. Think about the advice and exercises, and how they can have a fixed place in the patient's daily life.

Preventing Recurrence: An Action Plan

A characteristic of many health problems with which a physiotherapist is confronted in practice is the recurring nature of these problems. This often has to do with the connection between the health problem and things like an inactive lifestyle (lack of movement and therefore poor physical condition), certain habits (posture, smoking, etc.), stress, illness perceptions, and so on. Such connections should have been addressed during the analysis of the health problem or shortly afterwards, of course. Preferably, intervention is also targeted at this. However, not everything is equally easy to influence or change permanently.

That's why it's good to consider the possibility with the patient: What if you notice that your problems are recurring? What can you do? Together with the patient, you draw up an action plan or a first aid plan if recurrence is imminent or has occurred. You do this in the role of coach, so you stimulate the patient to come up with an action plan based on their successful experiences during the treatment process; where necessary, you provide the patient with additional tips.

An example of this sort of plan is:

- If I feel pain in my neck developing, I first check whether I am sufficiently relaxed while working;
- Furthermore, I will check whether I move sufficiently in between my working activities;
- If that doesn't resolve things, I also look at the quality of my sleep.

Focusing on posture, an example of this sort of plan is:

- When I notice that I have some stiffness or sometimes pain in my neck again, I ask myself the question: Does my neck pain have anything to do with my posture? Then I analyse my posture when I'm sitting at my desk.
- I analyse and correct my posture with the following three steps:
  - Am I positioned solidly on my chair? Can I feel my whole bottom, and can I feel the back of the chair?
  - Is my back being supported well by the backrest, and are my shoulders, neck, and back really relaxed?
  - Are my arms resting in a relaxed fashion on my desk and do I let myself 'drop down' properly onto my chair?
- Finally, I exercise my shoulders and neck every hour.

As a final example, we can look at an action plan to prevent recurrence that is focused on stress:

- If I notice that I become irritable, my sleep is affected, and/or I have a tense neck, then I analyse:
  - whether I include enough daily rest;
  - whether I keep some evenings each week free and then actively relax (instead of hanging out in front of the TV).
- If necessary, I take sufficient rest and do daily relaxation exercises for a few weeks.

Incidentally, bear in mind that all the elements from this example were experienced and 'discovered' by the patient earlier in the treatment process (goal: achieving sufficient relaxation).

It is often advisable to write down such an action plan because every person is inclined to forget such things, especially when things are going well and you have no complaints. The patient can keep the plan at home and refer to it if the situation arises.

Evaluating Collaboration

As a physiotherapist, you work closely together with your patient, often for fairly long periods of time. In order to strengthen the patient's self-management and autonomy and to be able to develop yourself as a professional, you can briefly evaluate this collaboration with each other. Especially with longer treatment processes, it is good to think about this. What went well, what went less well, what was helpful to the patient, what was not helpful, and did the patient feel adequately supported?

The following steps can help you with this process.

- Suggest to the patient that you want to evaluate your collaboration and ask them what they think of it. Say, for example, 'We worked together intensively to get you to recover well from your injury. I think it would be good to briefly think about this together. How did you experience our collaboration?'
- When the patient gives their view on your collaboration, you are actually receiving feedback from them. React by listening and considering what the other person means to say. Don't get angry or defensive! After all, you want the patient to be honest and tell you what they think is positive as well as negative. Ask if things are not clear. Take compliments, don't deflect them.
- Once the patient has given their view on your cooperation, it's your turn to do so. Reflect on your own role and give the patient feedback that they can use. If you're giving feedback, do it in the first person:
  - I see/hear that you...
  - I find that.../I feel that way...
  - I'd like you to...
- Finish your evaluation by giving a summary of this part of the conversation.

In Consultation

Open question	Before you leave...What do you take away from the treatment and guidance I've given you to prevent another injury?
	Um, well, I'm going to make sure that I bring enough variety into my workouts while exercising, and that I don't just do the same thing all the time. You particularly let me see and experience that I was training very repetitively. At the same time, exercising is now more fun.
Reflecting	That was an eye-opener for you to hold onto.
	Sure, that really helped me and it's going to keep helping me. I'm going to hold onto it!
Open question	What do you need to keep doing this?
	Well, not really anything, I guess. I mean, you've already given me tips on the internet and with the book. There are so many variations to use, I feel like I have more than enough!
	Excellent, excellent, good to hear!

THE PATIENT WANTS TO CONCLUDE THE TREATMENT PROCESS AND YOU DON'T (YET)

If the patient wants to conclude the treatment process and you don't (yet) want to, it is often because the patient is not satisfied; because the treatment goals have not, or only partially, been achieved; or they had different expectations. It is also possible that the patient is not satisfied with the relationship they have with you. It may happen that the patient does not show up for their next appointment. Then you're left with all sorts of questions. Maybe you think: 'I'm not going to try to find out; I'll wait for them to contact me—after all, it's their problem'. However, the patient's failure to show up may be due to all sorts of reasons, certainly including legitimate ones. It is therefore reasonable to make at least one attempt to re-establish contact. In the first instance, your goal is to find out what went wrong with the consultation and whether the patient wants to continue the treatment or not. If the patient wants to discontinue the treatment, you can then try to find out why and evaluate the treatment course together.

If the patient wants to end the treatment process, it would be best if they took the initiative and brought this up themselves, such as during the evaluation of goals and results at the beginning of a consultation. However, the patient may not always feel comfortable doing so. It is important to pay attention to this possibility and to be open to it. It is often quite a step for patients to bring something like this up, so make sure that 'your antennae' are on and that the patient feels free to take this step.

If the patient brings up wanting to end the treatment process, make an effort to find out the meaning of what they want to say. The patient is likely to find it difficult to say exactly what they think and will therefore express their opinion in veiled terms. Maybe they say, 'It doesn't bother me anymore—maybe it's still there, but it just doesn't cause me any more trouble', when in fact they mean, 'I don't believe the treatment will deliver any results'. Or maybe they say: 'Those exercises, I forget them far too often, so that's not going to work' while they mean, 'You are doing your best, and I don't give anything back. I don't want to do that to you'. By reflecting the patient's statement, you can help the conversation go much more smoothly because they feel understood. This allows you to find a more suitable solution with the patient.

Sometimes it happens that the patient wants to stop because they are seeing little or no result or because there are complications in the patient's view, while the physiotherapist thinks it is logical to not yet have a result and that there are no complications at all. Often, this can be explained by unrealistic illness perceptions and the patient's lack of knowledge. Try to avoid this situation by paying sufficient attention to education provision at an early stage of the treatment process, most likely during the first consultation (core task 4). And come back to this every now and then in follow-up consultations. If this situation does occur, show an interest in the patient's ideas and feelings regarding recovery (see also Section "Exploring illness perceptions" in Chapter 6). Then apply strategies to influence their illness perceptions (as described in Section "Giving advice" in Chapter 9).

YOU WANT TO CONCLUDE THE TREATMENT PROCESS AND THE PATIENT DOESN'T WANT TO (YET)

If you want to complete the treatment process and the patient doesn't want to (yet), it is usually because you and the patient have a difference of opinion about achieving the treatment goals. Based on your knowledge and experience, you can then see that stopping the treatment process is wise because you do not expect any further progress. How are you going to handle this?

If the Result Is the Reason for Stopping the Treatment

Naturally, you first evaluate the result of the treatment. Next, you and the patient enter the area of decision-making as discussed in Chapter 6. In the role of communicative detective, you offer various options to the patient (e.g. continue treatment, discontinue, or continue with modified treatment) and give the patient the opportunity to express their views on these options. The patient may also have certain options in mind. Then consider with the patient what chance they think there is for a result with the treatment. How does the patient see that and why do they see it like that? Check whether the patient is knowledgeable about this and explain it to them if this is not the case. In addition, consider your own assessment and how you arrive at that assessment. Also explain this so that the patient understands you. Further discuss the effort needed and/or side effects, as well as the pros and cons. Explore what the patient finds important and why, and discuss the different treatment options. Then come to a decision with the patient.

In short, your working method will be as follows (based on Chapter 6):

1 Evaluate the result of the treatment so far, in relation to the main goal;
2 Offer options: give up, continue, and other options;
3 Discuss opportunities, effort needed and/or side effects, pros and cons;
4 Check whether the patient has insight into the problem and the options with opportunities, effort needed and/or side effects, pros and cons;
5 Discuss and elicit values;
6 Make choices.

If you want to stop the treatment process because of complications and the patient doesn't want to (yet), the patient's level of knowledge is usually the reason: the patient does not interpret the symptoms as a complication or does not see the course as deviating, because they have too little knowledge about it. First examine what the patient already knows and then present those aspects which will give the patient increased insight. Then make a proposal for the follow-up, e.g. referral or examination (step 2), and go through steps 3 to 6 with the patient.

If the Relationship Is the Reason for Stopping

Another reason that you might want to end the treatment process when the patient doesn't (yet) can be due to the relationship. You may feel that your relationship with the patient is disrupted or that it is too weak to continue. However difficult this may be, it is crucial to discuss this with the patient and not simply ignore it. After all, a good relationship is the basis for effective assistance and without your role as confidant, you cannot work.

Start the conversation with the patient by saying that you have the feeling that there is something wrong with your relationship and asking how they see it. Leave the cause of the flawed relationship aside. Say, for example, 'I want to talk to you about something. I notice that we haven't really made a connection and that this prevents me from fully supporting you. How do you feel about this?' Or say, 'I've noticed that things aren't going so well between the two of us and I'm afraid that this will affect your treatment and recovery. How do you feel about our connection?' In these examples, pay attention to using the correct personal pronoun at the right time. Discuss with the patient how they experience your relationship and how they feel about it. Together you must find a solution to this problem. You may be able to make arrangements that will improve your relationship. Don't continue with a patient who says, 'Ah, we don't have to become friends. As long as you do your thing, then I'll do mine'. If a relationship of trust cannot be established, the treatment is doomed to fail. That's why it's also in the patient's best interest that you make a point of this.

Summary

In this last chapter of Part III, the end of the treatment process is discussed. The physiotherapist takes the role of communicative detective with regard to evaluating the treatment objectives and, in addition, employs the role of a coach on a regular basis. Three possible situations when ending treatment are discussed:

- The patient and you want to conclude the treatment process;
- The patient wants to conclude the treatment process and you don't (yet);
- You want to conclude the treatment process and the patient doesn't (yet).

If the patient and you want to conclude the treatment process, you evaluate the treatment result—you may consider having the patient work at home on treatment goals and/or preventing a recurrence and, if desired, you may evaluate the cooperation you have had. If the patient wants to complete the process and you don't (yet), this is usually because the patient sees the result as insufficient or because the patient does not experience their relationship with you as positive. It often happens in this case that the patient does not show up or cancels their appointment, making action on your part advisable. This allows you to find out what you can still do for the patient or to evaluate your relationship with the patient. If you want to end the process and the patient doesn't (yet), it is usually because you do not expect any further progress or because your relationship isn't good. You then find yourself in a situation that calls for shared decision-making, in which you can follow the same steps as discussed in Chapter 6. In any case, evaluate your collaboration and try to learn from it.

PART IV

If There Are Particularities

The competencies, skills, and techniques described in Part III of this book form the core of the physiotherapy discussion. However, there are times when these competencies are not sufficient for the situation. For example, in some instances, the conversation does not flow, or there is a complex situation where a sticking point plays a role. That's what this part's about.

Chapter 12 discusses problems in your relationship with the patient. Consider whether you connect with the patient—or just the opposite, with the relationship threatening to turn into a friendship. Chapter 13 elaborates on how to use communication in such a way that it improves the patient's motivation or strengthens their self-efficacy. Chapter 14 discusses self-management in situations in which the patient has reduced health literacy skills and how, as a physiotherapist, you can enter the patient's social context and see what influence this has on their self-management. In Chapter 15, you will learn more about pain and chronic pain, and especially about their consequences for the way in which the physiotherapist communicates. Chapter 16 is a short chapter that deals with the particularities in communicating with patients with anxiety and mood disorders. The conversation with special groups of patients is discussed in Chapter 17. These include conversations with children, (vulnerable) elderly people, and people from other cultures. Chapter 18 discusses special conversational situations and how to deal with them. These include conversations delivering bad news and 'risk communication'. Chapter 19 concludes Part IV of this book; it deals with conversations with the patient about potentially fraught themes such as stress and lifestyle.

The physiotherapy consultation

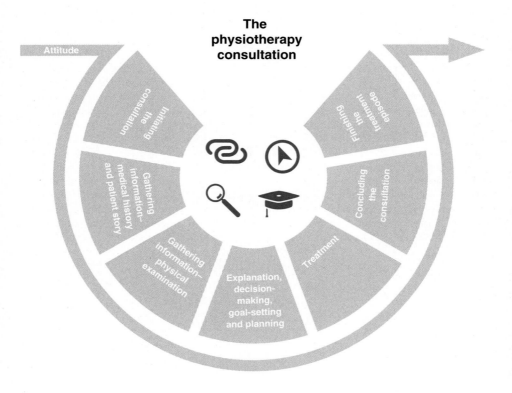

CHAPTER 12

Problems in the Professional Relationship

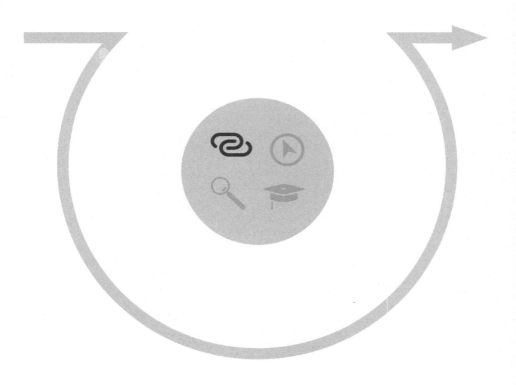

Every therapist realises how important the role of a confidant is for providing effective care. If something goes wrong in the professional relationship, which is only human, you want to respond adequately. In the following three situations, there is something wrong in the professional relationship:

- The relationship of trust between the physiotherapist and the patient is flawed;
- The relationship of trust becomes disturbed during the conversation: dissonance or friction arises;
- The physiotherapist and the patient develop such a good 'bond' with each other that the professionalism of the therapist is compromised.

These three situations each have different causes, as well as their own approach to being resolved.

THE RELATIONSHIP OF TRUST IS INSUFFICIENT

With some patients, you simply don't find the rapport you hope for. And even after doing hard work on the relationship, you still do not have enough connection to take on the role of confidant. Now what?

First of all, it may help to review Chapter 5, regarding the first impression and the first contact, as well as what is stated in Chapter 4 about building and maintaining the relationship with your patient. Did that all go well, or did you miss a few points there? In the latter case, it may be possible to 'repair' the relationship. Though it may not be as good as it would have been if everything had gone well from the start, you may yet be able to build a working connection.

To fix things, you need to look at how well you are attuned to the patient. Is there an adequate rapport (Dilts & Grinder, 1980)? Pay attention to body language, use of spoken language, speaking volume, and speaking speed. Attune yourself better to the patient than you did previously. It will probably deliver a result. If you are not yet satisfied, examine further why the relationship of trust between you and the patient got off to an inadequate start. Do you notice different interests, values which are too dissimilar, differences in personality, or differences in behavioural style? All are possible explanations. It may help if you come to understand where things are going wrong in your relationship; from this understanding you may come to a better attunement.

Besides attunement, your mindset can play a role. Do you notice that you're starting to annoy the patient? Do you feel a growing aversion to the patient? Watch out! Don't be guided by prejudice and don't focus on negative things. What you focus on tends to 'grow'. Realise that there is something good in every human being and that in every patient, there is an explanation to condone their behaviour. Let this be your primary mindset: discover what is good in the other and focus on that.

Finally, you may not have listened carefully enough or sufficiently enough to the patient, to what they *meant* to say. And you may not have shown clearly that you were listening, such as by reflecting. This in turn caused the patient to react in a certain way.

Eventually, with careful communication and practice, the group of people with whom you don't feel any 'chemistry' will be quite small. At this point, if you are not attuned to each other and are simply carrying on trying to force a relationship of trust, you will probably not have any clinical success, either. That's when it's time to propose continuing the diagnostics and/or treatment with a colleague. Don't make this suggestion too heavy and or too difficult. Say, for example, 'I'd like to discuss our way of working together with you. A good recovery requires that you and I work well together during your treatment. I have the feeling that our synergy is not working out well. How do you experience us working together?' Avoid looking for a culprit. Avoid hostility, even if the patient makes it difficult for you in this respect. If the patient feels the same, you can decide together that it is better for their recovery that a colleague takes over the treatment.

THE RELATIONSHIP OF TRUST DETERIORATES: DISSONANCE

Everyone knows this feeling: the conversation is going well, the patient and you are well attuned; in short, there is an adequate relationship of trust. Suddenly the conversation takes a turn that you don't expect. The patient becomes distanced from you, possibly even literally: the collaboration deteriorates and the conversation becomes awkward and difficult. If you're not careful, the mutual dialogue that you used to have changes into a discussion. You and your conversational partner don't seem to be able or willing to understand each other anymore.

What's going on here is called 'dissonance' in the relationship (Miller & Rollnick, 2012). In the past, the term 'resistance' was often used for this. However, 'resistance' implies blaming the patient, and that is not justified. The term 'dissonance' gives a good indication of what is really going on: the mutual cooperation is lacking, and harmony is absent.

Dissonance that persists is a threat to the relationship between the physiotherapist and the patient. Because the role of confidant is the basis for physiotherapy assistance, you have to take action.

Recognising Dissonance

Dissonance can manifest in several ways. You can recognise dissonance in yourself and your own behaviour. And you can recognise dissonance in the patient. Sometimes it's obvious that dissonance is the cause of the friction; other times not at all.

You can recognise dissonance in yourself by feeling uncomfortable, or by feelings of irritation or frustration. You may notice that you (constantly) have a tendency to interrupt the discussion, that you often say 'yes, but' in your head although you suppress it, or that you think to yourself, 'doesn't want to' or 'how stubborn!'. Incidentally, these thoughts prevent you from listening carefully to your patient. You can also recognise dissonance by physical signs of tension (in your abdomen, neck, or back, for example) or your cheeks flushing from the strain.

The patient's behaviour can also make it clear to you that there is dissonance. Such dissonance can be recognised by any one of the following reactions by the patient (Miller & Rollnick, 2012; Waddell & Sohal, 1998):

- **Defending:** the patient justifies their behaviour, including through accusing ('Well, if I had known more and had more information from the doctor, I would have been better off'), dismissing ('That's not so bad, it won't be because of that'), or defending ('I've been doing this for years, it can't be wrong').
- **Rejecting:** the patient shows that they see you as an opponent ('People like me know better').
- **Interrupting:** the patient keeps interrupting you.
- **Withdrawal:** the patient 'tunes out' by changing the course of the conversation.

An important criterion for identifying the above behaviour as dissonance is that the patient's behaviour changes quite suddenly.

Dealing Effectively With Dissonance

To reduce dissonance, you can do the following.

- **Take a step back:** Recognise the dissonance by naming what you yourself feel or think and/or what you think you see in the other person. Usually you have a reasonable idea of how this happened and what you did that caused the dissonance. Say, for example, 'I get the impression that I may be going too fast or saying something that you can't quite follow. Is that right?' Or 'I feel I sometimes have difficulty following you in things. Maybe you have that with me, too?'
- **Take a step sideways:** Examine where the dissonance comes from. Dissonance can arise on a variety of grounds. Think of the strongly divergent illness perceptions of the patient and the physiotherapist, or strongly divergent norms and values or attitudes. It may also be that the therapist wants to push a behavioural change more quickly than the patient can or wants. Finally, it could also be a misunderstanding: one of the conversation partners has not understood the meaning of a statement.
- **Moving forwards:** Try to restore the attunement between yourself and the patient in an appropriate manner, depending on the situation (see 'Think laterally'). Think about the further exchange of ideas/illness perceptions or a train of thought, explain relevant

norms/values, connect with the patient and their behavioural change if you have moved too quickly, explain your intentions, and test whether the patient can go along with this.

Although in many cases you will try to reduce dissonance in your patient relationships, it is not necessary to 'avoid' dissonance too frenetically and anxiously. Some cases or situations simply elicit some dissonance naturally. Above all, it is about keeping that dissonance manageable and trying to reduce it at an appropriate moment, thereby restoring the relationship of trust.

Some physiotherapists experience dissonance as a personal issue; they get the feeling that they have failed, that they are not nice or competent enough, and so on. It may then help to see dissonance as part of the communication process, something which is unavoidable in some situations. The communication process also says little about you as a person. It's because you're doing something that the patient *interprets* as not being 'in their best interest'. There's no direct cause for worry. Take action and take control.

THE BALANCE BETWEEN DISTANCE AND CLOSENESS IS DISTURBED

Sometimes your relationship with the patient becomes too personal and a kind of friendship develops. The patient trusts the physiotherapist so much that they discuss all sorts of private matters that have nothing to do with their health problem. Or the patient shares things with you that are related to the health problem, but are outside your area of competence. How does this happen? And how do you deal with it?

The concepts of 'distance' and 'closeness' take on extremes in the spectrum of the professional relationship that a physiotherapist enters into with a patient. A professional relationship has, as it were, two sides (Maes, Zotero). One side is that of distance and personal detachment, the other is that of closeness and personal involvement.

Distance is crucial in—among other things—applying techniques, methods, procedures, steps taken and/or treatment plans, determining whether physiotherapy treatment is indicated, and setting limits for the physiotherapy treatment. These are mainly instrumental rationality aspects, and distance provides overview, structure, and control. The roles of teacher and communicative detective need distance to function appropriately.

With closeness, your humanity is central. This involves creating and sharing meaning from within the personal relationship with the patient, through emotional and personal involvement. The physiotherapist must be sensitive to the patient's vulnerability. 'Being present' makes the patient feel understood and able to share their experiences (Baart, 2003; Hessel, 2009). Closeness is easily recognisable in the roles of confidant and coach.

Both distance and closeness are important in the professional relationship. To be able to provide solid assistance, it is essential to maintain both as much as possible. You'll then simply be more balanced. Sometimes you lean more to one side, sometimes more to the other. Maybe you even abandon one side for a very short time. But as soon as you do this for too long, the physiotherapy help you provide will no longer be professional.

The Closeness Becomes too Intense

A situation with too much closeness can arise if the patient feels the need to share personal things with someone because they have a poor social network. In the physiotherapist, they have found an empathic and respectful ear and whatever is preying on their mind has to be shared. Sometimes, the patient simply feels at ease and wants to tell their story. It is important that as a physiotherapist, you indicate what your competencies are and what they aren't. You may want to be a listening ear: indicate this and also say that you can't be more than a listening ear because you don't have the expertise to help the patient with their personal problem.

A situation with too much closeness can also arise if the therapist has shared personal information with the patient and the patient wants to start sharing personal information with the therapist as well. In this situation, the initiative largely lies with the therapist. Sharing personal experiences with the patient can be deployed professionally. The literature here speaks of 'self-disclosure' or 'selective self-disclosure' (Hill & Knox, 2001). In this case, as the word 'selective' suggests, a *specific* personal experience that you have had as a therapist is related to a professional goal: to prompt the patient to revisit the topic of conversation or the question asked. However, if you no longer discuss personal information with the patient selectively but in an unfocused and arbitrary manner, your professionalism is at risk: you become unbalanced and wobbly, because you are leaning too much towards the side of 'closeness'.

Getting too close to the patient cannot always be avoided—as a physiotherapist, you sometimes work closely with the patient for a longer period of time, and relationships often deepen or become more personal with increased exposure. The following focal points can help you maintain professionalism in the relationship with your patient.

- Prevent excessive closeness or inhibit it by only sharing personal experiences with the patient as long as this has a purpose within the framework of the physiotherapy treatment.
- Indicate what your expertise is and what it is not, by distinguishing between your professional role (musculoskeletal expert) and your compassionate role (a listening ear).
- If you ask questions about personal insights or private experiences, be clear about what you actually want to know and what you don't, and why it is important to talk about it (establish a connection with the patient's health problem).
- If you notice that the patient does not allow themselves to be guided by these interventions, give feedback in the first person and voice your opinion by saying, for example, *'I feel like you're entrusting me with things that you may regret later. I think it's better for both of us that we focus on the treatment'*, or *'You've entrusted me with things that are rather private. I don't feel very comfortable with this and I don't know how to deal with it. I'd like to focus on the exercises'*. Don't guide with hostility, but be quite clear. Non-verbal behaviour ultimately determines whether your message convinces or not!

Summary

Because the role of confidant is crucial for the deployment of the other roles, the quality of the relationship of trust with the patient must be sound. In this chapter, three problems are discussed in the professional relationship between the physiotherapist and the patient:

- The relationship of trust between the physiotherapist and the patient is flawed;
- The relationship of trust becomes disturbed during the conversation: there is dissonance;
- The physiotherapist and the patient develop such a good 'bond' with each other that the professionalism of the therapist is compromised.

If the relationship of trust between the physiotherapist and the patient does not get off to a good start, it is wise to invest in this again. Consciously make a better attunement with the patient and be aware of your own beliefs about the patient—the way in which you view them—and adapt them if necessary.

If there is dissonance in the relationship between the physiotherapist and the patient, it is important to reduce it, because dissonance threatens the cooperative relationship and therefore the quality of the care provided. Investing in the relationship of trust forms the basis for reducing dissonance.

If there is too much closeness between the physiotherapist and the patient, the professionalism of the support and of the professional is endangered. By looking at closeness and professionalism as two balanced sides of an equation, it becomes clear that the professional can only ignore one side for a short period of time. Professional support preferably takes place while keeping a balance between both sides: closeness and professional distance.

CHAPTER 13

Insufficient Motivation

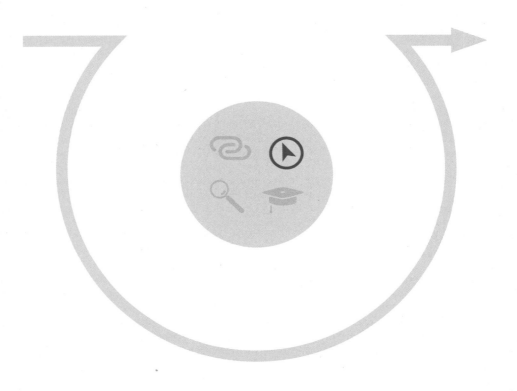

Being motivated and staying motivated is not easy. Patients often experience changing their existing behaviour as extremely difficult. And that's to say nothing of being able to maintain that behavioural change in the long term! Motivation plays an essential role in this, of course.

One of the reasons that behavioural change is difficult is the fact that almost everyone who has to and/or wants to change something experiences ambivalence in doing so. Ambivalence is formed by the patient's conflicting thoughts and feelings towards the change. These thoughts and feelings are about the pros and cons of the desired and current behaviour and also about the trust the patient has in being able to perform the new behaviour, seen as self-efficacy. If a patient is ambivalent, the arguments they give themselves for and against the change remain pretty balanced. The result, of course, is that the patient does not take action.

Motivational interviewing (Miller & Rollnick, 2012) is a style of conversation in which your conversation with the patient aims to reduce their ambivalence towards the change and thus strengthens the patient's inner or autonomous motivation. This is elaborated in The Section "Ambivalence" on the basis of the work of Miller and Rollnick (2012). Because self-efficacy has also been described and researched as an independent concept in the literature (Bandura, 2010; Picha & Howell, 2018; Rajati et al., 2014), a part of this chapter ("Reduced self-efficacy") has been devoted to it.

AMBIVALENCE

Ambivalent feelings and thoughts often form a barrier against the patient taking action, even if they have made a conscious decision about the treatment themselves or together with you (shared decision-making). The patient still struggles with the pros and cons of their decision. The consequence of this internal doubt is that they may not take action or may only maintain the desired change for a short time.

Ambivalence often gives the impression that the patient is not motivated. But it's too early to say. It is better to speak of a 'conflict' between the different interests that the patient experiences, thinks, and feels. Think of the objections and effort they have to make on the one hand and the change and results they long for on the other hand.

In order to help the patient 'overcome' their ambivalence, it is important, as a counsellor, to have a tolerant attitude and not to condemn the patient's ambivalence, but to see it as a logical aspect of change.

Ambivalence: An Internal Battle

The patient's statements make it clear that they are ambivalent. Although the patient mentions arguments and motivations which seem to be in favour of the change, they also mention things that argue against it, usually at the same time. The arguments and motivations in favour of the change are the disadvantages of the current situation and the advantages of the desired (new) situation. The arguments and motivations that argue against the change are precisely the advantages of the current situation and the disadvantages of the new situation. This creates four 'groups' in the arguments, feelings, and motivations of the patient. Figure 13.1 shows the ambivalence of the patient schematically.

Change Talk

The patient's statements about their ambivalent motivation partly argue in favour of the change. These self-motivating statements are called 'change talk': word usage that shows the patient's willingness to change. In your role as coach, you try to recognise, explore, and strengthen such change talk.

Change talk can be subdivided into preparatory change talk and mobilising change talk. Preparatory change talk consists of statements made by the patient showing their tendency

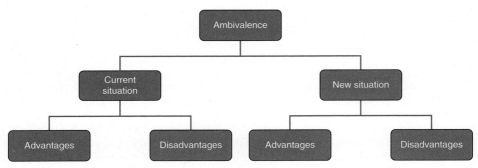

Figure 13.1 Ambivalence: the internal struggle for change.

towards changing, but not yet exhibiting a tendency to take action. This preparatory change talk can be subdivided into four types of statements:

- **Desires:** the patient says what they would like or what they long for. They articulate what they would therefore like to be able to do differently. For instance, 'I'd like to be able to go upstairs so I can sleep in my own bed'.
- **Reasons:** the patient says why they want to change. For example, 'I could do my own shopping again', or 'I could see my son's football match again'.
- **Abilities:** the patient expresses the extent to which they think that change is possible for/by them. This can be about the actual possibilities and skills a person thinks they need to change, but also about the confidence a person has in their chances of success. If the patient says something about their confidence, they say something about what is referred to in the literature as 'self-effectiveness' or 'self-efficacy' (see Section "Reduced self-efficacy"). Examples include: 'Well, these exercises aren't tricky, so I should be able to do that' and 'I don't know if I'm going to keep this up; I've had bad experiences with it'.
- **Need:** the patient indicates the urgency of the change, as in: 'I don't want anything half-baked any more, I really want to be done with it!'

As the patient's preparatory change talk becomes more articulate and robust, it becomes clear that their ambivalence towards the change is dissolving and their propensity for action is growing. The latter is also noticeable in the fact that in the end, another form of change talk is created: mobilising change talk.

Mobilising change talk indicates a propensity for action that can be recognised in three types of patient statements:

- **Commitment:** the patient uses words and phrases which indicate an intention or decision, as in: 'I'm going to do the best I can'.
- **Action:** the patient uses change talk in which an intention or movement towards action can be heard, such as, 'I'm going to do these exercises tomorrow' or 'I'm going to see this week how I like it if I go for a walk every night'.
- **Taking steps:** the patient identifies actions they have taken in preparation for change, such as, 'I've been to the gym to find out what it costs and what guidance they can give me when I go for a workout'.

The patient's statements in favour (or to the detriment) of the change are often about the more concrete and everyday things that are important to them. At this time, the patient is often speaking implicitly about their individual 'values': the things that are important to their existence. They might also be surfacing their feelings or beliefs. For example, hidden in the statement 'If I practise consistently, I will recover more quickly so that I can do my own shopping again' there can be the important value of 'independence' or 'autonomy' and the feeling of 'pride'. Thus, with their statements, the patient often implicitly reveals a 'deeper layer' of inner motivation.

Sustain Talk

In many conversations, change talk will be interspersed with statements by the patient in which they argue against the change. This is called 'sustain talk'. Sustain talk is often about the (implicit) advantages of the current situation and the disadvantages of the new situation. In the context of exploring the patient's ambivalence, you will also address this, in as far as it is strictly necessary.

Increasing Autonomous Motivation by Reducing Ambivalence

Ambivalence can be compared to an old-fashioned set of scales. The scales remain more or less in balance because change talk is on one side and sustain talk is on the other (Figure 13.2). In other words: the patient's inner motivations are balanced. Notably, the change talk doesn't weigh enough for the scales to tip to the side of active change.

Ambivalence can be reduced by coaching or guiding the patient. You can use the motto: 'What you pay attention to, grows'. In doing so, you connect with what the patient already says themselves: their sustain talk and change talk. You then guide the patient in the direction of change by paying more attention to the change talk, without ignoring the sustain talk. You do this at the patient's pace, not faster. You try to elicit more and more change talk from the patient, but without exerting pressure or trying to convince them.

Coaching the patient's motivation is done, for example, with open questions, reflections, and summaries. In doing so, you always try to connect with what the patient says about their motivation, simultaneously working in the direction of the change and the change talk. For example, you may ask the patient further questions about their change talk. As a coach, you react in a strategic way: you do not try to strengthen the sustain talk too much, such as by asking in-depth questions about it or by reflecting these repeatedly and/or firmly. Rather, you soften it by, for example, following up your simple reflection of the sustain talk with a reflection of the change talk that the patient has also used before. You also try to search for deeper layers in the patient's personal motivation by asking open questions about it or giving back reflections in which you carefully express this value to the patient (in order to make them 'think and feel').

Denying sustain talk or trying too hard to ignore it will usually result in the patient focusing more on the sustain talk in the conversation, with the result that it increases.

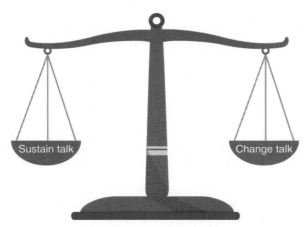

Figure 13.2 Ambivalence: the inner motivations of the patient are balanced.

Coaching by eliciting change talk is done on the basis of your role as confidant. In this role, you ensure that the patient feels free to say the things they want to say—both about sustaining as well as about changing. Only then does will change talk have real value as the patient's use of their change talk increases. In coaching, the patient's autonomy is central—their choice or wish is the deciding factor. So if the patient remains convinced that change is *not* desirable for them, despite your guidance, then you will have to accept this.

■ Levels of Reflection

Patients' statements about motivation are like an iceberg: one part is clear and lies above water, while a more important part lies underwater and is meaningful, without being named by the patient. Reflections identify the part of the meaning of the patient's statements that lies above as well as below the water. There are three levels of reflection:
- **Simple reflection:** names/repeats what the patient says (above the waterline);
- **Complex reflection:** identifies what the patient does not say but means (below the waterline);
In addition to these levels, the following forms of reflection are worthwhile tools.
- **Double-sided reflection:** identifies both sides of the ambivalence, both the sustain talk and the change talk. Important here is the sequence: it can be strategically useful to first reflect the sustain talk and finish off with change talk. This may weaken the sustain talk and focus the patient more on the change talk, reinforcing it.
- **Metaphors:** by reflecting with a metaphor, you can concisely give a name to a range of meanings. The use of a metaphor implicitly conveys a number of meanings without explicitly expressing them.
- **Reinforced reflection:** on the one hand, you connect to what the patient says; on the other hand, you formulate your reflection in a stimulating way that makes the patient think. Usually this means that you make your reflection exaggerated: much more forceful than what the patient said or meant or, conversely, much weaker. If you do this strategically or with some humour, you make the patient think.

Reducing Ambivalence Towards a Change

From your coaching role, you elicit the patient's motivations in a guiding conversational style. Eliciting begins with acknowledging what's there. You show that you understand what the patient is saying. It's even better if you can show that you understand what they *meant* to say. For this, empathic listening and the use of reflections are effective. The effect is that the patient feels understood. And by giving back to the patient what they say and/or mean, the patient gets an even better understanding of themselves.

Particularly in the case of the change talk, you can use reflections that put into words what the patient (also) wanted to say but (still) didn't say. A slightly different choice of words or a certain intonation can make all the difference. If the patient then recognises their motivation in what you give them back and responds to it with change talk, you guide them in the direction of the change.

In addition to reflections, you can use open questions focused on change talk. With these open questions, you explore the thoughts of change in breadth and depth. Think of questions in this area, such as 'Suppose you manage to exercise regularly and become more fit—what would that give you?' and 'It's better for your health, you say. What would it mean to you if you were healthier?' or 'How important is your health to you?' You can also explore the different types of change talk by asking open questions, as in: 'What are your reasons for doing the exercises on a regular basis?' (reasons) or 'How important is it for you to deal with this now?' (need).

A special way to use open questions is the use of 'scaled questions'. This technique allows you to investigate how important the patient thinks the change (e.g. the exercises or the advice) is.

For example, 'How important are these exercises to your recovery? Can you give it a number between 0 and 10, where a 0 stands for completely unimportant and a 10 for the most important thing there is?' If you then ask the patient to explain their grade, they'll typically use some change talk. Exploring this further by means of open questions and giving reflections often results in even more change talk. You can also ask: 'What makes you give a 4 and not a 2, for example? And what else?' Or 'What do you need to turn the 4 into a 5?' The effect may be that the change talk you elicit from the patient will increase the number. In general, higher grades are reasons to explore to what extent someone is ready to take steps to make lasting change.

Finally, you can use summary as a skill in guiding the patient towards change talk. In your summary, you list the patient's motivations. You do this strategically, by first summarising the patient's sustain talk and only then turning to the change talk. Incidentally, you apply such a summary less frequently than reflections.

Persuasion has no added value in reducing ambivalence. However, the patient may sometimes need specific information or lack certain knowledge; these gaps may contribute to them remaining ambivalent. Sharing and exchanging information can certainly be useful then. In this case, first ask the patient's permission to provide them with any relevant information, as well as to examine what they already know (see also Section "Sharing information" in Chapter 6). Then provide information and conclude with a stimulating open question, such as, 'What does this mean for your situation as far as you are concerned?'

In Consultation

	... For your knee problems, it would be good to do exercises that improve, among other things, the muscle strength of your thigh muscles. *Oh, does that really help?*
Reflecting	You doubt whether that's useful? *Well, um, yes, my knees are worn out anyway. So there's not much more to be done about that, is there?*
Reflecting, open question	Indeed, the exercises won't improve the osteoarthritis. What do you see as the cause of your knee pain? *Well, yes, so the osteoarthritis, my knees are worn out and there's not much one can do about it, except to get a new knee. And I'm not keen on that, at least for now.*
Reflecting, asking in-depth questions	You think your knee pain is caused by osteoarthritis. Do you think there are any other causes? *Well, no, not really.*
Asking permission	Maybe I can tell you something about that? *Yes, of course.*
Sharing information Open question	Osteoarthritis is known to lead to a decrease in muscle strength in the thighs, extensors, and flexors of your knee. This reduction in muscle strength in turn leads to you putting more strain on your knee joint and knee ligaments than necessary. And in your case, that most likely leads to pain. What do you think of that? *Mmm, makes sense. So you mean that exercises for the muscle strength in my thighs can eventually relieve the stress on my knee, so I have fewer problems?* That's right! *Only I'm not really good at doing exercises.*
Asking in-depth questions	Oh, tell me more? *Well, I often don't last very long and I'm not very disciplined and so on.*
Reflection on sustain talk	You don't expect to last long enough for it to take effect. *Yes. I surely have to do it longer than a couple of weeks, right?*
Giving information	Sure, you should preferably do the exercises for three months in a row.

Continued

In Consultation—cont'd

	Pfff, three months, that long!
Reflection on sustain talk/a closed question	Mmm, three months of exercises, you would not be keen. Are there other things you aren't keen on?
	Well, um, are there any fun exercises? Not so boring, I mean.
Reflection on change talk	It would make it easier for you if the exercises were fun to do.
	Yes, and not the same thing every time. So with some variation.
Reflecting/open question on change talk	Fun exercises and enough variation. I can help you with that, sure. Assuming this succeeds… what would you eventually like to get from the exercises?
	Well, less pain, more able to do things and able to walk further. That's what I'm hoping to achieve.
Asking in-depth questions	How long can you walk now?
	Well, half an hour tops!
Reflection on change talk	And you'd like to be able to walk much further without pain in your knee.
	Yes, my husband and I could go walking for three hours at a time! And on holidays, we often go into the mountains, so sometimes we would walk for five to six hours. But I don't see myself doing it just like that anymore.
Double-sided reflection	You don't see yourself walking all day anymore, and at the same time you are quietly hoping that with less pain in your knee, you could still go for long walks with your husband on your holidays.
	Yes, that would be great! Walking is the ultimate relaxation for us.
Reflection on change talk	Walking gives you a lot of relaxation. You really enjoy doing this together with your husband and that also makes it important to keep up the exercises for your knee for a longer period of time.
	Well, if I could. That would be lovely.
Summary (change talk – sustain talk – change talk)	Mmm, let me see if I can figure it out. You have indicated that you would like to get rid of the pain in your knee and that you would like to do exercises for it, but that in the past, you did not keep up such exercises for very long. What would help you is that the exercises are fun to do and contain enough variety. Your motivation to keep exercising is to be able to walk with your husband again for a few hours and finally to be able to go into the mountains together again for a whole day. Would you like to add any other points?
	Mmm, no, that's it. I'm actually curious about the exercises you have for me!

REDUCED SELF-EFFICACY

Self-efficacy indicates the degree of confidence a patient has in their own ability to perform certain actions at a specific point in time. In other words, it encapsulates the 'possibilities' the patient can envisage in changing themselves. This is expressed in the statements the patient makes about it: their change talk or sustain talk.

Self-efficacy is determined, among other things, by previous experiences of success or failure and the way in which the patient categorises these experiences, or to what factors the patient attributes their success or failure. Self-efficacy is an important predictor of behaviour that affects health or illness (Bandura, 1994, 2010). Low self-efficacy predicts a reduced chance of demonstrating the right (health) behaviour at the required time, such as doing daily exercises or following advice. In other words: if the patient has too little trust in their own abilities, it often results in ambivalence about their status quo, which is a good reason to give the matter explicit consideration here.

Exploring Self-Efficacy

The patient's self-efficacy is evident from their statements. Taking stock of this starts off by listening carefully to what the patient means to say. The statement 'Mmm, I don't know if that suits me' may indicate that the patient thinks they can't do it. This becomes clearer the moment the patient says, for example, 'I don't know if I'm going to be able to keep it up, you know!' Understanding what the patient means and reflecting on it or asking questions about it has often already given you a good idea of the patient's self-efficacy.

Working with scaled questions also offers possibilities here. You can ask the patient: 'How confident are you that you will do these four exercises three times a day, including once at work? Would you give it a number between 0 and 10, where 0 stands for "I don't feel confident about it" and 10 stands for "I'm sure I can do this".' As self-efficacy is very context-specific, it is very important that you describe the desired behaviour of your patient in a specific situation sufficiently and explicitly in your question. Low grading can be regarded as sustain talk, high grading as change talk. If the score is lower than 7, it is generally useful to spend more time reflecting further with your patient. Incidentally, giving a figure is not always necessary, as it is also possible to work more qualitatively and to ask the patient to express their confidence in their own abilities. You can also choose to use an intermediate form, such as: 'How confident are you that you will do these four exercises three times a day, including once at work? Do you have: no confidence, some confidence, moderate confidence, a lot of confidence, or a huge amount of confidence?'

If the patient's self-confidence is low, such as in 'a little confidence' or is, for example, grade 4, you continue the conversation to examine with the patient the reason for this: 'What makes you give yourself a 4?' This often provides starting points for solutions and/or opportunities for improving self-efficacy.

How to Use Communication to Improve Self-Efficacy

If a patient indicates low self-efficacy, there are several things you can do to help improve it. The essence of this is that you make the patient think and try to elicit change talk.

- Scaled questions are helpful in strengthening self-efficacy. For example, as a follow-up to the previous scaled question, ask: 'You give yourself a 4; why did you not give yourself a 2?' Or you might help the patient formulate a request for help by asking: 'What do you need to increase your confidence by 1 or 2 points?' A strongly eliciting and somewhat provocative approach may be needed when you notice low scores such as a 2 or a 3: 'I was thinking, I expected you to give yourself a 1'. Applied at the right time and with the right person, this can be effective and can trigger change talk.
- Patients sometimes see all kinds of obstacles and then get 'stuck' in their ambivalence. You help patients to look beyond such obstacles by using a special form of scaled question: 'Let's say we meet again in a week and then you give yourself a 6; what would have had to happen in the meantime?' Another way to look past obstacles is by asking: 'What would be a first possible step?' Or by looking for positive exceptions by asking the question: 'What possibilities do you see to really get going with it?'
- Some patients with low self-efficacy feel that they succeed at nothing and that they never have. The opposite is frequently the case: often situations can be found in which the patient is or has been successful. This may be the same sort of situation, but could also be a similar situation in a completely different field, such as work or a hobby. Ask, for example: 'Have you ever successfully changed the way you work?' And then continue with: 'How much confidence did you have in yourself back then?' and 'What made it all work out successfully?' By stimulating the patient to look at situations in which they did have confidence and were successful as well, their self-image is refined, creating a base for increasing their self-confidence in the current situation.
- Discovering traits in themselves which are helpful also has a positive effect on the patient's self-efficacy. Ask about it: 'Which of your personality traits do you think will help you in this?' and 'Could you give me an example of a situation where this trait has helped you?'

This immediately creates a possibility of being able to conform to such traits. This also strengthens self-confidence.

- By pointing out positive qualities to the patient, you as a therapist confirm that the patient can do it and also strengthen their self-efficacy. Say, for example: 'The care with which you proceed when you try to do this exercise will help you to do these exercises well and regularly at home'.

- Finally, searching for resources is useful. Think of getting help from others, using notes as reminders, or using an app on a smartphone. Social support can greatly enhance the patient's confidence in their success. Investigating together with the patient which resources are desired and available and how to use them may be necessary to enhance self-efficacy. Ask for support, for example: 'Who in your social circle can help you do this consistently?' Or ask for an example: 'Who do you know in your environment who is successful in doing exercises to treat certain problems?' and 'What could you learn from them in this regard?' In the Section "The social context" in Chapter 14, you can read more about how and when to make use of social support.

There are many more strategies available for improving self-efficacy. This section mainly describes the communication that takes place on self-efficacy. It certainly does not provide an exhaustive overview of strategies to improve self-efficacy.

Summary

In this chapter, the guiding role of the coach is described in relation to motivating the patient. Motivation cannot be imposed by the therapist. The act of persuasion can even be counterproductive because the patient is ambivalent—they think and feel that the advice, the treatment, or the exercises can be productive, but at the same time they also see the disadvantages, such as the effort they have to make. By helping a patient who is ambivalent to express their conflicting thoughts and feelings and become aware of them, the possibility of influencing them in the interests of the patient arises. To get the patient to use change talk instead of sustain talk is a central task of the therapist, and one in which they frequently use reflection. Change talk consists of preparatory change talk (patient statements that advocate change) and mobilising change talk (patient statements about concrete steps, actions, or commitment).

The concept of 'self-efficacy' is also developed. This is the patient's estimate of their own ability to exhibit specific behaviour at a particular point, such as doing exercises or following advice. This assessment is reflected in the patient's statements: their sustain and change talk. By getting the patient to use change talk with regard to the possibilities they see and feel, their 'self-efficacy' increases. You can do this in different ways, such as getting them to take a first step in the right direction, helping the patient to think of previous successes, asking them to think of helpful personality traits, and jointly searching for resources.

CHAPTER 14

Insufficient Self-Management

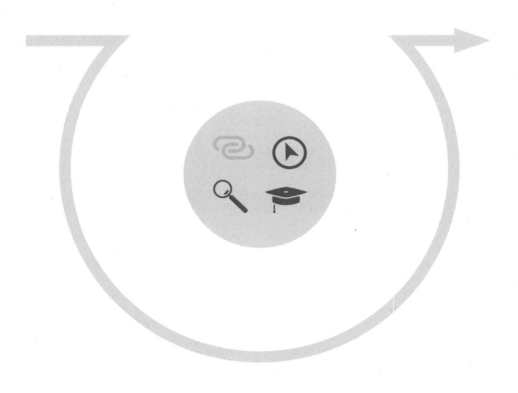

With professional communication, you want—among other things—to fully appeal to the patient's self-management skills so that their self-management is safeguarded and strengthened. For people with a chronic illness or disorder, self-management is understood to mean 'dealing with the illness/disease in such a way that fits in optimally with daily life' (*CBO, Zorgmodule Zelfmanagement 1.0,* 2014). Self-management in health problems of a transient nature is described in this book as 'the monitoring and positively influencing of one's own health problem by using one's own skills'. To engage in holistic self-management, the patient needs self-management skills in both cases. These are, among other things:

- the application of disease-specific knowledge and skills;
- self-efficacy;
- the capacity for self-development (Jedeloo & Weele, 2015);
- self-monitoring.

This chapter discusses two situations in which there is insufficient self-management. The first situation is one in which there is insufficient self-management because of reduced health literacy skills. In people with reduced health literacy skills, the ability to self-manage, make choices, and read and apply health information is moderately to strongly reduced. In order to better support this group of patients, it is of course important to adapt your way of communicating.

The level of health literacy skills varies widely across the EU and beyond. However, it is clear that even in economically prosperous countries, low levels of health literacy skills are common. For example, in EU countries, reduced health literacy skills which may be considered inadequate or problematic are seen at 29% (Netherlands) up to 62% (Bulgaria) (World Health Organisation, 2013). This picture is similar to countries outside the EU, such as the US and Australia (Australian Commission on Safety and Quality in Health Care, 2015; US Department of Health and Human Services Office of Disease Prevention and Health Promotion, 2010).

The second situation discussed in this chapter is the conversation with the patient about the way in which they are socially influenced and whether this influence helps them to achieve what they want to achieve. The relationship with self-management is explicitly made here. If the patient has poor self-management skills, then the importance of adequate social support increases greatly. This is further elaborated in Section "The social context" in Chapter 14, with consequences for communicative action in relation to the actualisation and use of effective social support.

REDUCED HEALTH LITERACY SKILLS

Health literacy skills are those skills that people need to be and/or stay healthy to cope well with their illness, through effective self-management. By definition, 'Health literacy skills are linked to literacy and encompass the knowledge, motivation, and competence of people to access, understand, assess, and apply health information in order to make decisions in everyday life and in relation to their own health, disease prevention, and health promotion in order to maintain or improve their quality of life throughout their lives' (World Health Organisation, 2013). The literature often describes three levels of health literacy skills (Jordan *et al.,* 2010):

- **Functional skills:** basic knowledge of health, the ability to read and write, the ability to understand information;
- **Interactive skills:** actively seeking information, asking for help, applying information to one's own situation and to new situations;
- **Critical skills:** being able to critically analyse and apply information in order to gain more control over one's own life.

Patients with limited health literacy skills are less able to acquire information, make value judgements, and take decisions regarding their health.

As a result of limited health literacy skills, people need more care, live unhealthier lives, have poorer self-management (including less therapy compliance, making errors in taking medication, and having a lower level of self-efficacy), and are less able to communicate with their care worker (World Health Organisation, 2013). Literacy, which forms part of functional skills, is an important basis for health literacy skills.

Recognising Reduced Health Literacy Skills

It is not always easy to recognise whether someone has reduced health literacy skills. The most important way to find out is by listening. Listen to what the patient means and not just what they are actually saying. Also, listen to their use of words, and to the sentence structures and length of sentences which the patient applies to their own verbal message. Often the wording is simple and the sentences are relatively short. Sometimes the sentences the patient uses are actually long yet unstructured, without 'full stops and commas, so to speak'. A patient describes their problems and symptoms in a simple way if their knowledge about them (i.e. functional skills) is limited. Moreover, their opinion about the health problem and its solution can be simple and unsubtle.

If you notice one or more of the following, you should watch out for reduced functional skills:
- The patient often arrives at the wrong time.
- The patient makes comments such as (*Toolkit Laaggeletterheid LHV*, 2015):
  - Sorry, I forgot my glasses.
  - Can you fill this out for me? My writing is so illegible.
  - Doctor, I forgot my reading glasses, can you tell me what it says?
  - I'll fill out that form at home.
  - I can't read because I'm word blind.
  - Those leaflets are so complicated.
- The patient did not complete the questionnaire.
- If you hand over a leaflet upside down, the patient does not automatically turn it over, but puts it away immediately.
- The patient asks 'for the usual way'.
- The patient repeatedly misunderstood and/or did not do the exercises properly.

Finally, you can explicitly and specifically examine whether a patient is illiterate by asking the following questions
- To what extent do you manage to fill in forms independently?
- How often does someone help you to read letters?
- How much do you understand information about your health?

Of course, you must precede such questions with an introduction in which you explain why you want to ask the questions. For example: 'I'd like you to fill in a paper questionnaire. That's why I'd like to take a brief look at how easy this is for you to do'. Incidentally, the three questions mentioned above have been formulated as open questions. Sometimes people with a low literacy level have difficulty with this technique and you may find it necessary to reformulate the questions as closed questions.

Limited health literacy skills due to problems with interactive and critical skills are more difficult to identify. Indications for this may include the following (partly overlapping with functional skills):
- The patient asks for 'the usual way'.
- The patient repeatedly misunderstood and/or did not do the exercises properly.
- The patient finds it difficult to summarise an explanation in their own words.
- The patient can't formulate their questions to you very well.
- The patient makes (repeated) comments such as:
  - Yes, the doctor's leaflet was so complicated.
  - No, I never read. Television gives me enough information.
  - Oh, I thought that the appointment was tomorrow.
- The patient does not give adequate answers if the question is complicated and/or long.

How to Communicate in Case of Reduced Health Literacy Skills

An important next step is to adapt your way of communicating to the reduced health literacy skills of the patient. A sharp distinction cannot be made here between adjustments for reduced functional skills, interactive skills, and critical skills. However, some adjustments in your communication may respond more to functional skills and others more to interactive or critical skills. Fundamentally, you need to adapt your vocabulary, the length of your sentences, and your sentence structures. You adjust only what is necessary so that the way you communicate resembles the way in which the patient communicates. Aim for optimal attunement.

The following focal points apply mainly to adjustments for reduced functional skills, but also partly to reduced interactive skills and to a lesser extent to reduced critical skills.

- Speak calmly.
- Use simple language and short sentences, but no 'baby talk'.
- Keep your introduction short.
- Give your explanation simply and concisely, without a lot of details.
- Structure the information and your conversations well; regularly point out the common theme to the patient. Say, for example: 'We know enough about your back now. I would like to talk to you now about how to maintain your health' or 'First I want to talk to you about what's bothering you' and later 'Now I'm going to present you with some treatment options'.
- Assume limited prior knowledge. Ask if the patient can explain what they know about the issue and then provide additional information.
- Keep the abstraction level low; do not use graphs and tables.
- Illustrate your explanation with just one or very few pictures if you can.
- Illustrate your explanation with experiences/feelings: let the patient do things, copy you, and feel a connection with what you have told them (if possible).
- Don't give too much of an explanation in one consultation: focus on the most important things and return to your explanation the next time.
- A leaflet usually does not help; it is often too complicated and just creates insecurity and fear.
- Make very limited use of comparisons. If you use a comparison, choose one that you can use more than once during the explanation; choose simple and strong 'frames' (see also Section "Giving advice" in Chapter 9). Beware of the risk that your comparison or metaphor will be taken literally.
- Use these steps in the (shared) decision-making about the treatment:
  - Explain what the patient has.
  - Explain what they can do about it (different possibilities).
  - Explain why it's important that they do this.
  - Make sure the patient understands.
  - Find out what the patient's preference is.
  - Come to a decision.
- Use the 'teachback method'. At the end, ask if the patient can recount it all by asking, 'Can you explain it in your own words?' or 'I've talked a lot, would you mind summing it up for me in your words?' or 'What I'm curious about is what you're going to tell your wife when you get home'.

THE SOCIAL CONTEXT

Health and health-related behaviour (e.g. lifestyle and therapy compliance) have a strong connection with the patient's social context. That is, the social context in which a person finds themselves partly determines their health. Human behaviour, such as following advice, doing exercises, expressing or indeed not expressing pain, lifestyle, and going to a physiotherapist or postponing it are all partly determined by how someone is influenced by or thinks about their environment (de Ridder & Schreurs, 2001).

A few examples to illustrate this:

- A child falls and hurts themselves. Does the concerned father or mother run directly to the child, or not? What do they say? 'Did you hurt yourself?'
- A man suddenly has severe back pain while working in the garden. Does his wife feel sorry for him and give him lots of attention? And what does she say to him? 'Do watch out, this is not good!' or 'Go for a long walk tomorrow and you'll be fine'.
- A middle-aged woman smokes and doesn't move around much. She'd actually like to quit smoking and get more exercise. When she brings it up with her family, they laugh at her: 'Haha, our mother in the gym! Don't worry, Mum, you're just naturally round!'

In the role of confidant, you pay attention to the social context of the patient in a consultation, so that you can better build and maintain a relationship of trust. In addition, for the roles of communicative detective and coach, it is important to understand the patient and their social context. Self-management skills are needed in jointly working out the treatment plan and its implementation. If the patient does not have enough of these skills, the social context will have a greater influence on their health behaviour. In other words, the extent to which the patient has to claim self-management skills in the therapy process determines the extent to which you, as a physiotherapist, respond to the social influence. In the next section, a 'decision scheme' has been worked out to support you in determining how far you should orientate yourself about the influence of the patient's social context in order to support the patient properly.

A Decision Scheme to Discuss the Social Context

Health problems are complicated, and it is precisely for this reason that patients generally consult a professional. As a professional, you know that health problems can be quite complex. The degree of complexity of the health problem often determines the extent to which the patient needs to assert their self-management skills. Health problems which are less complex require fewer self-management skills than those which are more complex. Based on this assumption, you could use Figure 14.1 as a decision scheme to determine the extent to which you orientate yourself on the influence of the patient's social context.

First, if solving the health problem requires fewer self-management skills on the part of the patient, the role of social influence is generally limited and your orientation may be brief. If, on the other hand, solving the health problem requires more self-management skills and if the patient only has these to a limited extent, then social influence is very important and you will need to examine this in depth. Third, the health problem may require a lot of self-management skills, which the patient may have to a great extent. The social influence will then be moderate. Of course, this is not a mathematical model; it tries to give an indication of the importance of self-management skills and the social influence, and therefore of the extent to which the physiotherapist will pay attention to social aspects of the health problem during the conversation.

Orientation on and Intervention of Social Influence

Depending on your assessment of the importance of the social influence, you will respond to this to a greater or lesser extent. In this conversation, you will initially be active as a communicative detective and later also as a coach.

Social influence can be split up into four aspects (Lak & Bijma, 2012):

- **Social norms:** what people consider to be normal or customary;
- **Social comparisons ('social modelling'):** upward (an example, 'I want to be like that'), lateral ('She is just like me'), and downward ('I do that better') comparisons with others;

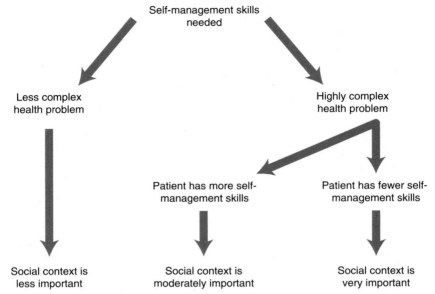

Figure 14.1 A decision-making aid showing the relationship between self-management skills and the social context.

- **Social identification:** the group to which people think they belong;
- **Social support:** the sources of support that people (can) have access to (companionable, emotional, instrumental, and informative).

Discussing Social Influence

In your discussion with the patient about these four aspects of social influence, the following question is central: To what extent is the social influence helpful in dealing with the health problem and/or can it be changed in such a way that it becomes helpful? Do the following:

- **Make an agenda or pick up on something:** Indicate that you want to talk to the patient about their environment and the extent to which this environment is supportive in achieving the treatment goals (such as exercising at home, exercising more every day, etc.). Find out to what extent the patient wants to discuss this topic with you. An alternative could be that you pick up on something the patient says at a certain point and use this as an entry to the conversation.
- **Gather information:** With the patient, explore the answer to the question: To what extent is your social environment and the way in which you are affected by this helping to solve your health problem?' Do this in the first instance by asking a more general question about it. In answering this question, you can then go into the four aspects of social influence so that the conversation becomes more solid and deeper: social norms, social comparisons, social identification, social support.
- **Discuss intervention(s):** Determine whether and on which aspect of social influence improvement is needed and what is feasible and what is not.

You can read more about the four aspects of social influence below.

Social Norms

When discussing social norms, you discuss the norms of the patient and the norms of their environment in relation to their health problem and health behaviour. What do they think about certain behaviour? What do they find normal to do for their health and what not? What are the advantages and disadvantages of these norms? Suitable questions for finding out include the following:

- What do you see as a healthy amount of daily exercise? What is normal for you in terms of…(e.g. daily exercise, healthy living, doing a good warm-up before sports, taking care of yourself in order to prevent injuries)? To what extent do you think that the amount of exercise you now have on a daily basis contributes to your recovery?
- What is normal for the people around you in terms of…? What do people around you think is a healthy amount of exercise? If you were to take more frequent exercise than your brothers and your parents, how would they react? How important is it to you if others think differently about this than you?
- To what extent do you see yourself doing these exercises daily, at work? How do you think you're going to react if others say anything?
- What do you think of doing the following daily…(e.g. sports, healthy eating, exercises to solve your complaints)?

Ultimately, you, along with the patient, want to gain insight into which norms help to achieve the desired behaviour and which inhibit it. If the patient realises that certain norms prevent or inhibit them from behaving in a certain way, you can help them by thinking together about how to change it.

Social Comparisons

With regard to social comparisons, you enter into a discussion with the patient about people they consider to be an example in relation to the intended behaviour (upward comparison). You can also talk about those people who the patient does not see as an example when it comes to the expected behaviour (downward comparison). In general, upward comparisons have a more positive effect on behaviour and behavioural change than downward comparisons (Lak & Bijma, 2012). It is therefore useful to confirm upward comparisons in particular. Lateral comparisons are literally and figuratively in the middle. Examples of questions you can ask to start the conversation include the following:

- Are there people from whom you can learn something about…?
- From whom could you learn things in terms of…(e.g. daily exercise, consistently following advice)? What can you learn from them?
- Who are you comparing yourself to as far as…?
- Who do you know in your environment who conscientiously/regularly does their exercises when there's something wrong with them? How do they do that?

Social Identification

Social identification is about determining the group with which the patient identifies with regard to their health problem, and about the extent to which the patient feels that they behave the same or would like to. There are two relevant possibilities in this respect (Lak & Bijma, 2012):

- The person thinks they behave in a certain way and therefore identify with a certain group (I exercise four to five times a week and am 67 years old, so I am a healthy older adult);
- The patient has a disease, disorder, and/or syndrome and identifies with the group of people with that disease, disorder, and/or syndrome (I am a COPD patient; I am a chronic pain patient), with the possible consequence that the patient will also act according to this identity and will probably find it more difficult to change their behaviour.

Examples of questions you can ask the patient if you want to discuss the aspect of social identification include the following:

- Which group do you identify with? Which group do you want to belong to?
- To what extent do you let your health problem determine what you do and don't do?
- What does it mean to you to be a heart patient?

- What does having diabetes mean to your life? To what extent does the fact that you have diabetes determine what you do and don't do?
- Do you know any other…patients? What similarities do you have with them? What makes you different from them? In which way do you not want to be like her?

The main purpose of this is to gain insight. It is then useful to consider along with the patient what they can do with this insight. Identifying with the group of people who have their disease, disorder, and/or syndrome can lead the patient to demonstrate behaviour that is unfavourable to the progression of the disease, such as inactivity. If this is the case, it is helpful to discuss this with the patient to find out if they see any changes they like, and if the ambivalence which they are likely to be feeling can be influenced.

Social Support
The last aspect to discuss with the patient is the social support they can appeal to, and/or which they experience. Social support consists of four different sources of support: companionable, emotional, instrumental, and informative (Sarason, 2013). In the case of companionable social support, the relationship with the other person exists because of the intended goal towards which the patient wants to work. If the patient's goal is to adopt a more active lifestyle, think of other athletes at a sports club, or think of a colleague who has the same complaints as the patient and also wants to follow advice and do exercise. Emotional social support means care, attention, and understanding from others in the patient's environment. Instrumental social support consists of tools of a material nature to support specific behaviour, such as getting a message on a smartphone to help remind someone of something. Last but not least, informative social support is about generic information about the patient's health, such as an information leaflet about the patient's disease.

Examples of questions you can ask if you want to discuss social support with the patient include:

- From whom (or what) do you have support in dealing with your illness, disorder, and/or syndrome?
- Who could support you to…?
- What does your partner have to do to help you? How can you discuss that with them?
- How can you be reminded to do your exercises more often?
- What would make you do your exercises three times a day?
- What information do you need to take exercise more often and sit around less often?

This approach provides insight into the level of social support to which the patient is entitled and to which they have access.

Summary

Effective communication appeals to, secures, and enhances the patient's self-management skills. With reduced health literacy skills, self-management skills are also reduced. Reduced health literacy skills require you to thoughtfully adapt your way of communicating. Accurate attunement to the patient's language level is important in the case of poor functional skills. If the patient uses simple language, the physiotherapist must adapt to this accordingly, such as by using short sentences and simple words from the patient's vocabulary, giving only a certain amount of information, and consistently using the feedback method for information transfer.

The extent to which self-management skills are required is often related to the complexity of a health problem. When a great deal of self-management skills are needed but the patient does not have them, the importance of discussing the social influence increases. The discussion with the patient about their social influences addresses the main question: To what extent are the patient's social influences helpful in solving their health problem and what can the patient do with this? Four sub-themes can support and actualise the discussion: social norms (the extent to which the patient wants their behaviour to depend on what others think and believe), social comparisons (who the patient uses as an example with regard to the desired behaviour), social identification (to what extent the patient identifies with a specific group and how their behaviour depends on this), and social support (what help does the patient think they need and how do they want to mobilise it).

CHAPTER 15

Pain

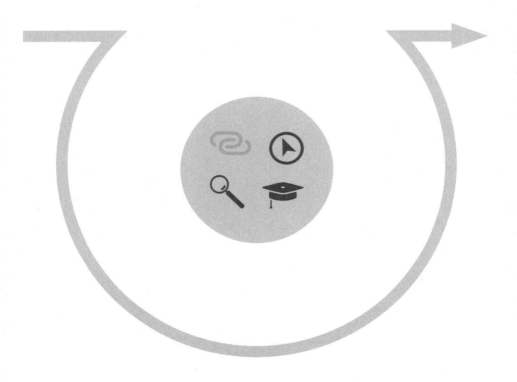

In many of the conversations that physiotherapists have with their patients, pain is an important theme—in fact, in primary care, this is probably key for half of patients (Koes *et al.*; Vos *et al.*, 2012). Because pain evokes all kinds of thoughts and feelings in the patient and this in turn results in certain behaviour, this chapter deals intensively with this matter. The patient's thoughts about the pain they are experiencing are strongly influenced by the people around them, and by the practitioner(s) with whom they come into contact. The patient will make an effort to communicate what they think and feel about their pain to the physiotherapist. The 'pain language' used by the patient and the 'pain language' used by the physiotherapist together constitute the first topic in this chapter.

Next we deal with the role of the communicative detective. As a communicative detective, you immerse yourself in some of the patient's illness perceptions. Together with the patient, you try to discover whether their thoughts and feelings about the pain are helping or actually hindering, in the sense that the behaviour elicited by these illness perceptions prevents or promotes recovery. You also analyse through the conversation (in the case of persistent or chronic pain symptoms) whether there is any central sensitisation. Central sensitisation consists of a generalised sensitivity of the central nervous system to nocisensory (pain) information.

Lastly, we will further explore the role of teacher and coach with regard to influencing the patient's illness perceptions and to structured pain neuroscience education.

HAVING A CONVERSATION WITH A PATIENT ABOUT PAIN

Talking to the patient about pain is a complex process. For example, the words used by the patient and the therapist, as well as the non-verbal support or language they use, are significant. They implicitly reveal a lot about each person's perceptions of pain and the health problem. These perceptions, in turn, are important for the behaviour of the patient and the therapist alike. It's good to think about this in a general sense before moving onto chronic pain.

The Patient's Pain Language

When patients want to describe their pain, they often use phrases such as 'sharp or cutting', 'oppressive or squeezing', 'as if a nerve is being pinched', 'enough to make me go crazy', or 'it's stuck'. From this, we can see that people look for words that describe how they *experience* their pain. At the same time, they look for words that match what they feel and think about their pain.

The words the patient uses, their *pain language,* are metaphors for their perceptions (Lakoff & Johnson, 1980, 2003; Munday *et al.*, 2019): for what they think, feel, and experience. The complicated thing is that, in one instance, the patient searches for and uses words to express the actual image of their pain, as in 'I think I have a hernia'. And in the other instance, they try to put more of their feelings and experience of the pain into words, as in 'it's stuck'.

To unravel the language of pain, listening well is your most important 'tool': empathic listening. You want to try to understand what the patient means and to help the patient express this by using reflections. With these reflections, you help the patient to express their feelings and the image they have of themselves. The non-verbal expressions used by the patient can help you to better understand and decipher the patient's statements. In addition, you use open and closed questions to seek clarification. Because the physiotherapist's reflections and questions help to clarify the patient's illness perceptions, you can also gain insight into the extent to which these determine the patient's behaviour in a negative or positive sense.

A second focal point in the patient's 'pain language' is the pronoun that the patient uses for the injured part of their body. Does the patient say '*my* leg' and '*my* neck' or '*that* leg' and '*that* neck'? In the last two examples, the patient themselves from their injured body part to a greater or lesser extent. With the words 'that leg' and 'that neck', the patient may implicitly indicate that they no longer see their leg and neck as a part of their body but experience them as a 'detached object'. The patient probably does this, typically subconsciously, because they no longer have control over the pain in the affected area. It may also indicate that the patient tends to take less responsibility for their health problem. Make sure that by listening attentively, you get more of these implicit messages. And keep talking consistently about *'your'* leg' and *'your'* neck'. Do not participate in the patient's use of distancing language.

In Consultation

	I have terrible pain in this area (pointing at their bottom, at the height of the sacroiliac joint). Sometimes when I stand up, it's like a sudden stabbing pain! (their eyes get bigger when they say this)
Reflecting	Then the pain is really intense.
	Yes, huge. It makes me catch my breath. It must be a nerve I feel there.
Reflecting	The pain is so intense, it makes you think of a nerve.
	Yes, it has to be! It doesn't feel like it's just a muscle.
Open question	Mmm, mmm. Where else do you feel the pain?
	Well, something in my lower back.
Open question	And how is your leg?
	I don't feel anything there, no.

Nocebo, Placebo, and the Language of the Physiotherapist

Clearly, the words the patient uses to describe their health problem say something about their (illness) perceptions and about their behaviour. In addition, the words you use as a physiotherapist also contain (illness) perceptions: your own. Hopefully these are helpful perceptions, but it is possible that through your choice of words you are also—subconsciously and unintentionally—transmitting negative or obstructive illness perceptions to the patient. Think of statements such as: 'it's stuck', 'we'll loosen that up', 'that's (not) right', 'you have bad posture', 'your back is worn out', 'your pelvis is twisted'. Or think of metaphors such as 'It's like a hinge that needs to be oiled' in order to explain the usefulness of mobilisation or manipulation to a patient. And, of course, non-verbal communication plays an important role here: your facial expression, emphasis, hand gestures, and so on. In the literature, clumsy or negative terminology is called 'nocebo' language which causes a 'nocebo' effect (Evers *et al.*, 2018).

It seems that patients derive an important part of their illness perceptions from what care workers tell them (Darlow *et al.*, 2013). This relates to not only positive but, unfortunately, also negative images and perceptions. By paying attention to your own 'nocebo' vocabulary and avoiding this, you may be able to prevent strong negative illness perceptions in your patients.

In addition to the nocebo effect mentioned above, the placebo effect also plays a role here (Testa & Rossettini, 2016). With regard to your use of words, this means that you create a positive expectation through the words you use. Think of saying things like 'My impression is that you are fit and ready for training; that will certainly help you recover from this problem', 'Your neck and shoulders seem strong to me' and 'Although I can see that your back pain is really stressing you, I also get the impression that your back is strong and robust. It's known that we rarely damage our backs; at the moment, nothing is damaged in your back either'.

In concrete terms, this means that in the first instance, if you do not yet know what the patient's health problem is, such as during an initial consultation, it is wise to choose neutral concepts and words. You are curious and interested in the patient's illness perceptions and explore these through reflections and (open) questions. As you become more familiar with the patient's health problem, you can become more specific in the terms you use with them. In any case, it is important to be aware of the meaning of the words you use and of the fact that this meaning is partly determined by how the patient listens to you and in what context you say things. That may sound like you're walking on eggshells—and sometimes you may be. As a physiotherapist, you should develop your vocabulary with the nocebo and placebo effects in mind.

THE COMMUNICATIVE DETECTIVE AND PAIN

In patients with persistent or chronic pain, the communicative detective identifies all the consequences—cognitive, behavioural and physical, emotional, and social—and integrates these into an explanatory model unique to the patient (Caneiro *et al.*, 2017; Nijs, 2011; O'Sullivan *et al.*, 2018). From this model, the therapist shapes the therapy approach along with the patient. This approach is very much in line with the working method in core tasks 2 and 3, as described in Part III (Chapters 6 and 7). Working with a dialogue model can provide excellent guidance in this respect. Because cognitive, behavioural and physical, emotional, and social consequences have already been discussed in other chapters, the next section will only give an assessment of central sensitisation, focusing on enumerating the illness perceptions in patients with chronic pain.

Of course, in order to list these effectively, the role of the confidant must be guaranteed. This sounds easier than it is. People with persistent or chronic pain symptoms are often tense and are not always given enough sympathy and time to tell their story. This may mean that you have to work harder, and possibly need more time, to build a good relationship of trust. So make sure you pay enough attention, as well as keeping communication consistent. Attune yourself to the patient, take your time, stimulate them to share their thoughts and feelings with you, and help them to do so.

You'll want to make a joint agenda at the beginning of the conversation: discuss broadly what you want to do and what you are looking for, then ask the patient to indicate what they want. Next, decide together on a procedure for the first consultation. In this way, the patient becomes more involved and your analysis will be better.

Then you can start your work as a communicative detective in core task 2. It's especially important now to pay attention to starting off your actual interview. The patient should feel as if they have an invitation to tell their personal story. Peter O'Sullivan, researcher and expert in persistent pain, gives an inspiring example. He often starts the conversation with 'Tell me your story'.

Exploring Illness Perceptions

We already discussed the basics of exploring and discussing the patient's illness perceptions in Chapter 6. To repeat the points:

- Stay consistently in the role of confidant.
- Listen really well. Listen both to what the patient says and what it seems they want to say. Use open questions and reflections to further clarify things.
- Try to connect to what the patient has already said about their beliefs, whether intentionally or by chance in their comments. Ask in-depth questions and reflect.
- If the above is unsuccessful or insufficient, ask explicit questions about the patient's illness perceptions. You will find many possibilities and examples for this in the Question Lexicon on Evolve.
- Discuss whether the patient's thoughts are also accompanied by negative emotions. Think of them feeling tense, worrying about the pain or recovery, being sad, feeling sad, giving up trust, etc.

As a communicative detective, as soon as the patient's illness perceptions become clearer, you also try to jointly examine the patient's behaviour. How does the patient behave, what do they do and, indeed, not do as a result of their pain? And is their behaviour in line with their beliefs of what is going on, or do you discover discrepancies in this?

Explore the patient's behaviour by asking questions about what they do or don't do with the part of their body which is in pain. Some examples include: 'What do you do when you're in pain?', 'What do you think is happening at that moment?' and 'What is it (e.g. "lying down") that improves your pain?' If you discover (or think you see) discrepancies, ask the patient about them or mention your observation to them. Take note: safeguard your relationship of trust now by paying extra attention to your warm and empathic non-verbal communication! For example, you could ask in the first instance: 'To what extent does what you do if you're in a lot of pain relate to what you think is going on?' If you find that this doesn't elicit anything much, then name the discrepancy you think you see: 'You said earlier that you don't expect to have broken anything in your back. At the same time, I hear you say that you are going to lie down to spare your back and let it recover. How do those two statements tie together?' Try to conduct this conversation with sympathy and reflections. Humour could also come in handy here.

Gathering Information on Central Sensitisation

To orientate yourself on the presence or absence of central sensitisation, you can follow two strategies. Of course, combinations are also possible. Central sensitisation is defined as 'an increased responsiveness of nociceptors in the central nervous system to either normal or sub-threshold afferent input' (Louw *et al*, 2011 & 2017).

In the first instance, it is possible to latch onto the patient's story. This means that you ask further questions about any signs and symptoms of central sensitisation when the patient mentions it themselves. This makes the conversation more natural: you use the opening in the conversation offered to you by the patient.

In the second instance, you can bring up the subject yourself. It is often advisable to first inform the patient about the purpose of the questions you want to ask. The patient's willingness to think along with you and to answer your questions increases with the insight you give them. You could, for example, say: 'Because of your prolonged head and neck pain, you may have become more sensitive to things like light, sound, and pain in general. This happens more often in people who suffer from prolonged head and/or neck pain. Now, if you don't mind, I'm going to ask you a few questions to get a better idea of this'. Next, you examine the various phenomena associated with central sensitisation.

THE ROLE OF TEACHER AND COACH IN THE CASE OF PAIN

The common thread in this book is that in both the diagnostic phase—while taking the history and during the physical examination—as well as in the therapy phase, the patient must be well informed. This means they are informed about what is going to happen, what is going on, why certain questions are important, what is expected of them, why a certain exercise is good to do, and so on. This is no different in the case of acute, persistent, or chronic pain. It is up to the patient to determine how valuable they find this information and to what extent they allow themselves to be influenced by it. The information you provide to the patient supports the diagnostic process by making it possible to discuss topics, helping the patient to think along with you, reducing the chance of dissonance between patient and physiotherapist, making it possible to discuss personal topics, and so on. Moreover, it helps the patient make a decision about the treatment.

In almost every situation, but certainly with chronic pain, it is necessary to inform the patient in the diagnostic process about, among other things, the influence of their thoughts on their behaviour, the sustaining role that their own behaviour could play in their complaints, the (understandable) 'interpretation error' that the patient may make regarding the nature and cause of their pain (e.g. pain is not the same as damage or harm), and the possible hypersensitivity of their nervous system (central sensitisation). Without this insight, it is virtually impossible to arrive at an adequate and shared decision regarding the treatment plan. This insight and the subsequent shared decision-making also form the basis for the patient's motivation for therapy interventions, such as pain education provision and a behavioural approach.

There is a difference between informing the patient and providing education to the patient. Informing is aimed at increasing the patient's knowledge; this is the role of the communicative detective in the diagnostic process or the role of the teacher in the therapy process. Education supplements the information that the acquired knowledge should lead to a change in the patient's behaviour. In providing education, you enact a combination of the roles of teacher and coach. Education provision almost always takes place in the therapy process.

Influencing Illness Perceptions About Pain

Influencing patients' illness perceptions is not an easy task. It demands a lot from the therapist: their patience, their knowledge, and their skills.

The communication strategy most commonly used to influence patient perceptions is to provide education. Other strategies, however, are also effective. In this section, several of these strategies are described separately. But because these strategies are complementary to each other, they are usually used side by side and interchangeably in everyday practice (Bunzli *et al.*, 2017).

In Section "Giving advice" in Chapter 9, we explored the difference between implicit and explicit learning in patient education and how this is linked to the level of misconceptions the patient may have. This classification of misconceptions about illness perceptions is also very useful in pain education provision. As a reminder, we identified misconceptions:

- **based on lack of knowledge:** 'my calf is still sensitive when I just try rolling out my foot' (a patient with 'muscle shortening' after their tear of the gastrocnemius muscle has recovered in a shortened position; they don't understand what's going on);
- **based on a false concept:** 'pain is always a sign of damage';
- **based on several false concepts:** 'my shoulder is worn out and therefore I'm in pain';
- **on the basis of a set of coherent false concepts (paradigm):** 'I have a bad back, it's in the family; I will always be in pain'.

Figure 15.1 shows these misconceptions in a diagram, thereby providing a rule of thumb for pain education provision. The idea behind the diagram is that simple and knowledge-related misconceptions can often be very much influenced by explicit knowledge transfer, or explicit learning. Misconceptions that conceal a comprehensive system of views on pain and the patient's health problem, as is usually the case with chronic pain, are better influenced by implicit learning.

Examples of explicit learning in education provision include:

- **Explicit explanation of information:** 'I've examined your back and can't find any abnormalities. So you can use your back and move as normal. That will even do you good. Exercise is a tremendous aid to recovery'.

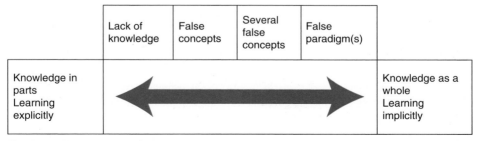

Figure 15.1 Education provision about pain: the connection between the patient's misconceptions on the one hand, and learning and education provision on the other.

- **Providing alternative information:** 'In 90% of cases, acute back pain like yours goes away within six weeks without the need for treatment'.
- **Connecting with existing knowledge:** 'You told me earlier that when you have back pain, you often use heat to aid recovery. The tense muscles in your neck will probably respond well to this'.

Examples of implicit learning in education provision include:

- **Using metaphors:** 'Bending over is like going skiing again after a long time. In the beginning, it takes some getting used to and it's a bit difficult, but you can still do it. Within an hour, you're on top of it again. That's the way it will be for your back: the more you do it, the better it's going to be'.
- **Experiencing it tangibly:** 'How does it feel when you bend over? What difference do you notice between the first few times you bent over and now? You were expecting more pain. What do you think about that now?'
- **Making a comparison:** 'You're worried about the creaking in your neck. The following could possibly help you: Could you make a fist? Now move your wrist. Do you hear the crackling sound? Now relax your hand and move your wrist again....Indeed, the crackling sound has gone. I think the creaking in your neck also has to do with muscle tension—in this case, of your neck muscles. If the muscle tension in your neck decreases, the creaking will also decrease, I expect'.

Chronic pain often involves a false paradigm regarding pain and the patient's pain-related symptoms. In this case, influencing the patient's illness perceptions will often be a complex and lengthy process, in which the patient may exhibit ambivalence with regard to what has been learned. The patient's learning process then probably takes a lot of time and needs to be tackled in a structured way. Also, due to the ambivalence of the patient, you and the patient will probably need a great deal of patients. As the physiotherapist, you should try to elicit change talk from the patient in relation to the message. To this end, next we will look further at structured and systematic pain neuroscience education provision.

In Consultation

Open question	What do you think of my explanation so far? *Mmm, well, so you're saying the pain I'm feeling is there, but it's actually much less strong than I'm feeling right now because my pain system is too active...so there's no damage which is causing the pain?*
Sharing information	Your pain is real and present. At the same time, it's a false alarm in the sense that nothing is broken. *But what they've seen on the pictures of my back, that shows that there's something wrong, doesn't it?*
Reflecting	You expect the abnormalities seen on the X-ray of your back to explain your symptoms. *Yes, of course!*
Reflecting Asking permission (sharing information)	Indeed, it does sound so logical that an abnormality on an X-ray gives an explanation for the problems you are experiencing. May I show you a study in which they analysed MRI scans of people with no back problems? *Yes, yes, sure.*
Sharing information (data)	So in this study, people without back pain were given an MRI scan. The results are shown in this Table (*see* Table 15.1).

In Consultation—cont'd

	One of the things shown by your X-ray was a supposed narrowing of the intervertebral disc. From the table, you can see that in people of your age (42 years), such a narrowing occurs in almost half of the people without back problems.
	So those people aren't bothered by it?
	Correct.
	Mmm, pretty remarkable.
Reflecting	Yes, remarkable, and at the same time actually quite common. You
Using metaphors	would see changes like these on an X-ray just as you would see the crow's feet around your eyes.
	You mean it's just part of getting older?!
	Yes, exactly.
Providing additional	In addition, six months ago, you had no problems with your back,
information	while it is unlikely that your X-ray looked very different then.
	No, that's true, okay.
Open question	What do you think of my explanation of your pain system and that you are more sensitive than normal to pain?
	Well, it makes sense. I get it, too, although I've never heard of it before. I also find it hard to accept…
Reflecting/open question	It's new to you and it's hard for you to fully fathom it. What do you think could help you with that?
	Well, to know what it means for me, what I can do about it.
	……

A second way to influence illness perceptions is to go along with the patient's rationale and then modify it. You make use of the fact that the patient's illness perceptions are often the result of their own reasoning pattern and the connections they ascribe to it. During your conversation with the patient, the central question is how the patient thinks their pain originates. While the patient works out their rationale, you state why, in your opinion, you think this is no longer

TABLE 15.1 ■ **Age Related Prevalence of Degenerative Changes in the Spine on an MRI in Asymptomatic Subjects***

	Age (yr)						
Imaging Finding	**20**	**30**	**40**	**50**	**60**	**70**	**80**
Disk degeneration	37%	52%	68%	80%	88%	93%	96%
Disk signal loss	17%	33%	54%	73%	86%	94%	97%
Disk height loss	24%	34%	45%	56%	67%	76%	84%
Disk bulge	30%	40%	50%	60%	69%	77%	84%
Disk protrusion	29%	31%	33%	36%	38%	40%	43%
Annular fissure	19%	20%	22%	23%	25%	27%	29%
Facet degeneration	4%	9%	18%	32%	50%	69%	83%
Spondylolisthesis	3%	5%	8%	14%	23%	35%	50%

(Source: Brinjikji et al., 2015).
*Prevalence rates estimated with a generalised linear mixed-effects model for the age-specific prevalence estimate (binomial outcome) clustering on study and adjusting for the midpoint of each reported age interval of the study.

correct. You can also ask questions about this to let the patient discover their 'reasoning error' for themselves. Do this in a calm and non-confrontational tone. Once the 'flaw' is visible, the patient has room to 'fix' it with an alternative line of reasoning based on new or different knowledge that you give them.

The great advantage of this working method is that you get to understand most of the patient's knowledge and beliefs. You only introduce 'new knowledge' to a limited extent, which means the change remains relatively small for the patient. This also makes the change more fluid for the patient and usually results in less ambivalence.

In Consultation

	...are you sure it's not a nerve, then? That's how it really feels!
Reflecting	The fact that it has nothing to do with a nerve actually surprises you. *Yes.*
Asking permission	Mmm, maybe we can figure out how you came to your conclusion and how I came to mine. Then that might explain why we arrive at different conclusions. Is that an idea? *Mm, yes, that's okay...*
Closed (encouraging) question	Could you try to put it into words why you think there's something wrong with a nerve? *Um, yes. I'm trying...when I make certain movements, I suddenly feel a shooting pain. It's, uh, it's like there's a nerve that's being pinched. It's also a very intense and stabbing pain.*
Reflecting	Okay, so it's the intensity of the pain that makes you think of a nerve, is that right? *Yes, exactly. I've never felt it this acute before.*
Reflecting	I think I get it. Because the pain is so intense and sharp, you associate it with a nerve that is being pinched or something. Because, of course, a nerve is very sensitive. Is it like that? *Yes, exactly!*
Asking permission	Then may I explain to you how I've come to a different conclusion? *Mmm.*
Explaining	Well, if something goes wrong with a nerve, we always notice it because of the way it radiates or spreads. And the clearest signal for such a situation is radiation into your lower leg and eventually also tingling in your lower leg. And you don't have that. *Yes, that's right, I don't.*
Explaining	Besides, in the area where you have pain, right at the top of your buttock, there is no nerve pathway that could get trapped or anything. So the pain you feel can't come from a nerve. How does that sound to you? *Oh! I didn't know that...I would really say I feel a nerve there, but according to you, that's not possible...*
Reflecting	You have to get used to the idea. *Yes, yes...and so the pain I feel in my bottom has something to do with a muscle.*
Explaining	Yes, that's the most logical explanation. When I look at where you have the most pain, I certainly come to the conclusion that it is indeed a muscle. *Mmm, well, okay.*

Patients regularly have a purely physical explanation for their pain. This often causes problems when imaging diagnostics are used. Structural damage is then 'fatal' in the patient's view: this causes them to have complaints and they will hang onto them as long as there is damage. Especially with diagnoses such as osteoarthritis and rotator-cuff ruptures, insurmountable situations arise, because these are types of damage in which repair, in the sense of repairing the cartilage or the rupture, is not possible. The following strategy may offer a solution in situations such as these.

This strategy consists of education provision. By providing education, you disconnect the shape from the function. You do this by explaining to the patient that the *shape*, the thinner layer of cartilage or the ruptured part of the rotator cuff, does not necessarily have to have consequences for the *function* of the body part in question. Explain that as a physiotherapist, your main expertise is in examining and treating the function and not so much in determining whether there is something wrong with the shape (other experts are good at that!). Because it is almost always possible to improve the function of a muscle, joint, tendon, etc. with exercises, the therapy approach should be aimed at this.

A metaphor may make this clearer. When you buy a new pair of shoes, the shoes are very nice and not worn out in any way. Still, they often take a long time to feel comfortable. What's more, well-used shoes sometimes seem to be badly worn out, but are actually very comfortable to walk in! With our bodies, it is often the same: if abnormalities are found, this certainly does not immediately mean that something is malfunctioning or can't be fixed.

A final method to influence the patient's illness perceptions is known in the literature as the Socratic style (Siemonsma *et al.*, 2013). In a Socratic conversation, you try to 'challenge' the patient's ideas and beliefs with regard to their pain. When you challenge their beliefs, you do so in a sincere, supportive, and enquiring way. By doing so, you and the patient try to investigate to what extent their thoughts, feelings, and behaviours are useful/useless, correct/incorrect, complete/incomplete, helpful/obstructive, and/or sustainable/unsustainable. A key here is that you don't challenge the patient themselves—just their perceptions and ideas. The patient should not feel challenged and interrogated as a person. Therefore, closely monitor your role as a confidant. It can now also be helpful to ask 'permission' by saying: 'May I challenge your thoughts and feelings about your pain a little? I wonder if they are correct and whether they're helping you to get closer to your goal'.

If you apply the Socratic method, you use three tools to challenge the thoughts, feelings, and behaviours of the patient:

- Questions for clarification;
- Questions to test thoughts, feelings, and behaviour;
- Hypothetical questions that place the problem in a new perspective.

Questions to clarify beliefs mainly examine what the patient is trying to say, what they think and feel when they say something, or what they imagine in concrete terms. For instance, you might say: 'You said it feels like your neck is totally stuck right now. I'm curious and wonder what you mean by that. Could you explain it to me?' or 'You have a slipped disc. Tell me what you think that looks like?'

When you use questions for testing, you try to see whether a thought, feeling, or pattern of behaviour is useful and helpful or actually doing the opposite. You do this by asking questions such as: 'Is this a fact, a suspicion, or an estimate of yours?' or 'To what extent are you sure that's what's going on?'

In hypothetical questions which place the problem in a new perspective, you search with the patient for new interpretations of their pain, and hope that these will then create new illness perceptions. For example, you could ask the following: 'You say your neck feels like it's stuck again. To what extent is that the full picture?', 'You say that you have a slipped disc again. What could be an alternative explanation for your symptoms?', 'Suppose your pain lessens and the image of your back remains unchanged; what makes you have fewer symptoms?', or 'The orthopaedic surgeon said that your neck shows a lot of wear and tear. To what extent did the surgeon possibly mean this as a metaphor?'

During the Socratic conversation, your intonation and non-verbal behaviour are extremely important. With these aspects, you convey the intention behind your question. Make sure your intention comes across as warm, compassionate, supportive, and sincere with each of your questions for the patient. In addition, respond to the patient by regularly reflecting on what they said or meant. Preferably do this before you ask your next question. This guarantees your role as a confidant.

Finally, there are two points which have already been mentioned in Section "Providing education" but which are important not to lose sight of. Keep in mind that the education you provide must be understandable and memorable. And help the patient to be open to the questions you ask them or education you provide by asking their permission to do so at the appropriate times.

Structured Pain Neuroscience Education Provision

If you focus on concepts and paradigms about pain in a patient with chronic pain, you must proceed systematically. A step-by-step plan as published by Nijs (2011) or an approach as published by Moseley and Butler (2013) is useful, and research supports this (Nijs *et al.*, 2014). The aim of this step-by-step plan is to change the patient's illness perceptions in order to eventually achieve an effective way of coping—that is, changing their behaviour. Although it focuses on changing beliefs and paradigms about pain, the plan uses an explicit form of learning. This is because the structure of the step-by-step plan is based on the knowledge and facts which you ultimately want to transfer to the patient in order to bring about a paradigm change. However, the knowledge you want to transfer is also accompanied by a lot of implicit learning through the use of examples, metaphors, and the patient's experience during, for example, exercise.

Topics covered in pain neuroscience education (PNE) provision are: the cause of the pain, acute versus chronic pain, how to influence pain, and the factors which maintain chronic pain (Nijs, 2011). The following step-by-step plan can support PNE provision (Nijs, 2011).

- **Step 1:** Explain what the useful function of pain is (protection) and what the differences are between acute pain and chronic pain. Pain always takes priority, even if it is a false alarm.
- **Step 2:** Explain the nervous system: the central nervous system with spinal cord and brain; the peripheral nervous system with an enormous number of nerve cells with nerve fibres; sensors on the nerve fibres, with different functions (thermal, mechanical, chemical); and activation of the sensor and therefore the transport of a stimulus via the nerve fibre to the spinal cord, if the stimulus is strong enough.
- **Step 3:** Explain how the processing of a stimulus takes place. After activation of the nerve fibre, the message or signal goes to the spinal cord. The spinal cord connects to other nerve fibres that run to the brain, among other things. Chemical processes transmit a signal from one nerve cell to another. The combination of certain chemicals causes transmission of the signal; other combinations do not.
- **Step 4:** Explain the role of the brain in whether or not it transmits information or messages from one nerve fibre to another, all connected to each other in the spinal cord. The brain is a volume control for the information that enters the spinal cord: it amplifies the signal, weakens it, or keeps it constant. For example: if you start paying attention to the sound of an air conditioner, you will notice it more and it will bother you more.
- **Step 5:** Explain that there is no fixed relationship between damage and pain. The human body's natural analgesic system is up to 60 times stronger than any medication for pain. Sometimes there is a lot of damage and little pain, as with a footballer who wants to finish an important game. Sometimes there is little damage and a lot of pain, such as a loose bit of skin on your cuticle that irritates you enormously and that you are aware of all the time.
- **Step 6:** Explain that the brain continually filters the enormous flow of information that comes in based on thoughts, emotions, memories, and primary motives. Explain the 'pain memory' ('no brain – no pain') and the relationship with the duration of pain (persistent

or not). Pain memory works in the same way that you recognise words: you don't read all the letters separately and one by one, but rather you see the word as a whole, even if certain letters don't match; you quickly overlook them. The same goes for the pain memory: it fills in the information that you think is there.

- **Step 7:** Explain that sensors adapt to the number of signals they receive. In this case, the number of sensors increases, increasing the sensitivity to pain. This is just like how the sensitisation in the fingertips improves when someone learns to read Braille.
- **Step 8:** Explain central sensitisation: harmless messages are amplified and are thus considered dangerous. The pain system can be compared to an alarm system. In the case of central sensitisation, the alarm system is set too sensitively.
- **Step 9:** Explain that the pain memory in the brain is so well developed or 'trained' that it has a stronger effect than in people without chronic pain. If you have felt pain in a certain area very often, you have become practiced in feeling pain. You're then more likely to feel pain, even when there's no danger.
- **Step 10:** Summarise—stimuli from tissues pass through sensitive sensors via the nerve fibres to the spinal cord; there, the signal is amplified by the volume control, which is 'on', and it continues to the brain, where the 'trained' pain memory is easily activated.
- **Step 11:** Discuss why this is happening to the patient and establish connections with what has been learned, causes, thoughts, the sensitivity of the pain system, and the pain memory.
- **Step 12:** Apply what has been learned in follow-up consultations, exercises, homework assignments, and so on.

This step-by-step plan is a guideline from which you can deviate as soon as you consider it desirable. If you succeed in making pain education provision truly personal, i.e. attuned to the level and experience of the patient, this will give the patient a lot of insight. Apart from the usual ways in which attunement takes place, you construct it, especially in the examples and metaphors you use. These have to be taken on board by the patient.

Finally, education provision is an interactive and creative process. Because of the interaction between you and the patient, the education you provide will be better and more tailored to their unique needs (Watson *et al.*, 2019). By starting with a question to the patient at every step and on every subject, you involve them in the education process. You call up existing knowledge and thus have the opportunity to connect directly with what the patient already knows. Ask the patient to recount what you have explained on a regular basis. This greatly increases the effectiveness of the education. Pay further attention to the relationship of trust during your conversation. The concepts you offer the patient often differ wildly from their current ideas and thoughts about pain, and there is a potential for dissonance (in your relationship). By regularly asking the patient what their thoughts are and by reflecting their answers, you can often prevent this from happening.

Don't forget: the patient will most likely be ambivalent about the message you are giving them. This is logical, given its complexity and the fact that patients have a different paradigm for pain. Be patient and maintain the relationship of trust you have with the patient. Coach the patient in their ambivalence, help them put it into words, and help them to understand and accept the new information about their pain. By making PNE provision interactive, you contribute to this shift. Furthermore, you try to prompt change talk, aimed at getting the patient to accept the new concept of pain.

Summary

The patient often expresses their illness perceptions regarding pain by describing their experience or their perception of the pain. You can use reflections, among other things, to clarify their pain language. This gives you both a clearer idea of the patient's beliefs about their health problem. The physiotherapist's pain language also conveys their own perceptions of pain to the patient. Therefore, accuracy in the physiotherapist's own language is essential.

Chronic pain is a therapeutic challenge, especially on the communicative level. Because of the complexity of chronic pain, extensive neuroscience education provision can be helpful, preferably using a combination of explicit learning and implicit learning, such as through the use of metaphors which would appeal to the patient. At the same time, it remains essential to maintain sufficient interaction and an exchange in communication, which is not always easy. The role of confidant may come under pressure, not least because the new concepts provided are often far removed from the knowledge and concepts that the patient has always used. In the role of coach, you can help the patient to overcome their ambivalence towards the new information.

CHAPTER 16

Patients with Mental Health Conditions

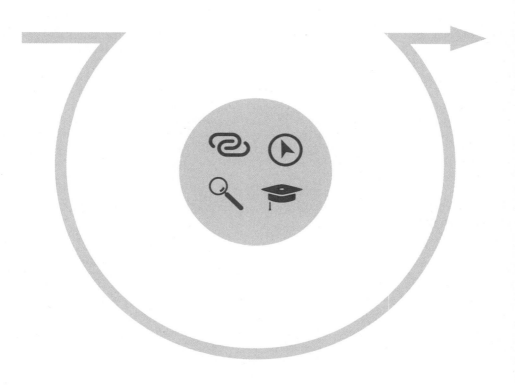

Common mental health conditions include mood (such as depression and mania) and anxiety disorders. It is estimated that 27% of the European population (prevalence in just one year) endure mental suffering which affects their daily functioning (Wittchen & Jacobi, 2005). Nervous exhaustion and burnout are also common.

Let's look at some concrete data on this problematic situation (Kessler *et al.*, 2009; Statista, 2018; Van Zwieten *et al.*, 2014; Schaufeli, 2018):

- Anxiety disorders (that is, being anxious without any real threat) occur in 8% of the world's population.
- Depression occurs in 6% of the world's population.
- Nervous exhaustion is a state of mind in which a person can no longer relax sufficiently, resulting in physical complaints (e.g. palpitations, high blood pressure, muscle pain, headaches) and mental complaints (e.g. restlessness, emotional blunting, loss of interest, irritability).
- This is also the case with burnout, but here the symptoms are often more severe and there is emotional exhaustion, depersonalisation, and inability to perform in work and family life. Moreover, the cause of a burnout is different than in a case of nervous exhaustion—it is linked specifically to work-related stressors. Amongst employees in the European Union, 10% score high on a burnout scale; percentages differ greatly from country to country (from 4.3% in Finland to 20.6% in Slovenia).

A health condition in the patient regularly leads to ineffective behaviour and thus adversely affects the course of the health problem for which the patient is consulting the physiotherapist. Of course, it is important that as a physiotherapist, you are aware of the fact that your patient has a mental health condition. Noticing early warning signs of a burgeoning mental health condition can also be important.

IN CONVERSATION WITH PATIENTS WITH ANXIETY AND MOOD DISORDERS

If a patient has a mental health condition, this has consequences for your interactions together. In this chapter, you will learn about the focal points for communication with patients with the most common psychological disorders, i.e. anxiety and mood disorders.

How to Communicate in the Case of Anxiety and Mood Disorders

Some rules of thumb are given here for dealing with patients with anxiety and/or mood disorders. When applying these, it is important to always consider the context. Sometimes a rule of thumb applies more to one patient than to another.

The feelings and thoughts that the patient has and that are associated with (and characteristic of) their mental health condition often seem unreal to an outsider. But in fact, they are not. It is important to realise that the patient's thoughts and feelings in this situation are part of an illness or syndrome. As a result, these thoughts and feelings are much more difficult to explain than, for example, illness perceptions. The patient wants to get rid of these thoughts and feelings, but can't control them—and that's exactly what makes them mentally ill! The consequence of this is that as a physiotherapist, you must not try to refute the patient's feelings and thoughts, but rather accept them. Furthermore, it is advisable that in your interactions, you take adequate account of the patient's depressive and/or anxious thoughts and feelings.

Mood Disorders

A mood disorder is defined as a disturbed mood over a longer period of time. Think of persistent gloominess, mild to severe depression, or bipolar disorder. In the latter condition, the person's mood varies greatly: one moment sombre or depressed, the next moment manic (e.g. evincing excessive joy, anger, hyperactivity).

A mood disorder can easily be compared to a broken car engine starter. The patient is willing, but can't. For your interaction with the patient, this provides a number of necessary focal points:

- Be authentic and positive, but not overly cheerful.
- Compliment the patient if you can.
- Set small goals together with the patient.
- Stimulate the patient to come up with their own solutions and give them support (coaching or guidance).
- Don't be light-hearted about things the patient experiences as a serious problem.
- For things that are obvious, do not ask the patient whether they want to do it, but implicitly assume that they do and influence them on the 'what' and 'how'.
- Assume that you will receive little appreciation for your efforts. Don't let this affect your motivation; the patient would like it to be different, too.

Anxiety Disorders

Patients with an anxiety disorder suffer from unreasonable and morbid emotions. The anxiety has no real basis and in social terms, it causes the patient all kinds of problems. Anxiety can be generalised (generalised anxiety disorder, panic disorder), but can also be related to a past event (post-traumatic stress disorder) or a specific situation in daily life (such as phobias of spiders, social phobia, or fear regarding exercise).

Much of what the patient undertakes is from the perspective of their fear and the associated thoughts that 'it will all go wrong'. They are probably constantly trying to tell themselves that this is not the case, but an important part of the problem is that doing so doesn't work.

When working with a patient struggling with anxiety, it is worthwhile to pay attention to the following things in your contact with them:

- Take a calm, encouraging attitude that inspires confidence.
- *Don't* say: 'It's not that bad' or 'There's nothing to be afraid of'.
- Ask what you can do to reduce anxiety, for example by changing the context.
- Acknowledge the fear, but don't dwell on it too much or for too long.
- Together with the patient, decide on a goal and an approach and support the patient in this (their fear may cause them 'to be at a loss on how to proceed').
- Set low targets and confer on what the patient feels ready for.
- Keep everything organised, tackle it step by step, don't talk too much, and clearly state what you expect from the patient.
- Offer distraction—for instance, talk to the patient about things that interest them.
- Reinforce the desired behaviour where possible (and avoid sounding 'childish or patronising').
- Repeat things regularly because it is unlikely that much of the information will get through, at least the first time.

Summary

Patients with psychopathological disorders regularly visit the physiotherapist. This can make communication difficult. Taking the patient's thoughts and feelings seriously forms the basis for your communication. At the same time, as a physiotherapist, it is generally not meaningful to dwell on the patient's mental state for too long.

CHAPTER 17

In Conversation with Certain Groups

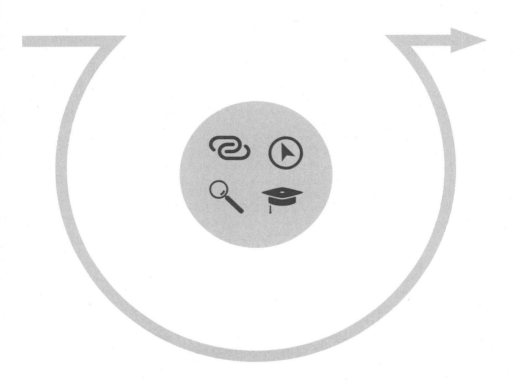

Every physiotherapist comes into contact with patients from all segments of society, from different backgrounds, with different cultural backgrounds and different ethnic roots, of different ages, and so on. Patients are part of (sub)groups in society and this may involve particularities in a communicative sense. This chapter is about working with such individuals: what you are doing differently to what you were doing before (as described in Parts I, II, and III).

The first theme to address is 'intercultural communication', a concept that stands for communication with people who have different habits and values than that of the care worker. The cultural background of the different inhabitants of a country can vary greatly. A city like Amsterdam, for example, has a population of more than 800,000 people from 180 different cultural backgrounds ("Gemeente Amsterdam. Onderzoek, Informatie en Statistiek", 2014). In a city like London, up to 300 different languages are spoken (*London*, 2020). This gives rise to a number of focal points for communication with patients; we discuss these in this chapter.

In this chapter, you will also learn about interacting with children, the elderly, and the mentally disabled. Finally, auditory and visual disabilities are briefly discussed, along with the focal points that apply here.

INTERCULTURAL COMMUNICATION

Many physiotherapists perceive intercultural communication as a complicated theme. In fact, intercultural communication *is* a strange concept, because it is not really about communication between cultures. Once again, this is about communication between people. And people are, by definition, different—sometimes a great deal, sometimes very little. The art of conversation is always to find attunement so that a partnership can be established here.

The view on intercultural communication in this book is partly based on the TOPOI model (Hofman, 2013) and the CCC model (Teal & Street, 2009). The TOPOI model distinguishes five areas of cultural differences and misunderstandings: tongue (language), order (relativity of truth), person (communication on a relational level), organisation, and intentions and influence (communication on a behavioural level) (TOPOI). CCC stands for 'culturally competent communication' and describes five essential communication skills and four critical elements to develop these skills.

Communication Between People From Different Cultures

In order to gain insight into what intercultural communication is, it is first relevant to consider the concept of culture itself. Culture can be seen as 'the common world of meanings' of a particular group or collective. This 'common world' consists of four parts that are often intertwined.

- **Language:** Each collective has its own language. For example, professionals often use jargon among themselves, and people from a certain region of a country often speak a dialect. In the language or dialect that people speak, you often recognise (implicitly) the knowledge and values and norms of a collective.
- **Knowledge, views, and images:** A collective has a common amount of everyday knowledge: opening times for shops, the rights and duties of citizens, the role of government, and so on. In addition, a collective has shared views on the social role of men and women, education, health, work and leisure, and so on.
- **Values and standards:** Values are things the collective finds valuable and important for that collective. Standards are rules or guidelines for acting in everyday social intercourse. A standard connects the value (what one finds important) with the behaviour in everyday life. One value, for example, is honesty, and the standard that can go with it is that you may not steal.
- **Symbols, rituals, and heroes:** Symbols are certain words, gestures, or objects that have a specific meaning for the collective. Think of certain clothes, a common hand gesture, or a

flag. Rituals are all kinds of activities that, in social intercourse, give expression to one's own group and cannot be separated from it. Think of a holiday, the way in which people greet each other, and ceremonies. Finally, heroes are the behavioural models within a collective: leaders, stars, idols, or martyrs.

The Link Between Language, Knowledge, Values and Norms

Let's look at an example to make a few things clear. The Inuit know about 20 different words for snow (it's a myth, by the way, that they have more than 200 words for snow). Their language thus offers the Inuit nuances for the knowledge they have about snow and what they want to be able to express about it to others and themselves. So if an Inuit asks an English person what kind of snow has fallen, the English person will quickly react in the following way: 'Well, normal, just snow!' An English person knows practically no nuances for snow. They are not relevant in English culture, there is little knowledge about it, and the English language does not allow them to express themselves in a nuanced way about it. Now suppose an English person goes to Alaska, lives there, and learns Inuit. They will need a lot of time to get to know and use the language nuances in Inuit. They'll never speak Inuit as well as an Inuit does. Therefore, even after a few years, the English person will most likely only answer the question of what type of snow has fallen (in faulty Inuit, of course): 'Um, just, uh, snow, uh, a little powdery'. The English person has insufficient knowledge of the language, true, but also lacks the underlying knowledge needed to understand the nuance and to understand that this nuance is really important.

Language, knowledge, and values and norms are strongly connected. In the example, therefore, there is not only a language problem, but also a knowledge problem and a different appreciation of certain things (values/standards). A similar situation arises when a Turkish patient with a poor command of English is asked by the physiotherapist to name the kind of pain they are in. The patient probably doesn't know all the nuances of pain that the physiotherapist knows and may not have mastered the English language enough to express these different nuances. So the patient's reaction could well be: 'Pain, yes, yes. A lot of pain'. The physiotherapist will interpret this as they always interpret the statements of their patients—as a nuanced statement—which is totally incorrect. And for the Turkish patient, this statement is also nuanced, as they think they have adequately indicated just how much pain they are in.

The Common World of a Collective

At the beginning of this section, culture was defined as 'the common world of meanings' of a particular group or collective. But how common is this world? And does that mean it's homogeneous? No, not at all. That may seem obvious, but we often assume this implicitly, frequently in the form of stereotypes. For example, 'all Chinese people work hard in their restaurants'. Or 'all English people like horse racing' and 'all Scots wear a kilt'. And so on and so forth.

No, to be homogeneous and communal are relative concepts within collectives. Even within a collective, new subgroups can be identified, for example 'loitering Scottish youth' or 'free-runners in London'. And these subgroups are also far from homogeneous.

People Are What They Are

Figure 17.1 (Hofman, 2013) shows how we should approach intercultural communication. The figure tries to depict three young people from different cultures, all of whom grew up in Great Britain. A is of Indonesian descent, B was born in the Congo, and C is a native English person from the Cotswolds. The most important principle is that all three have the same human nature, with the same basic universal needs (food, shelter, sexuality, security/safety, and acknowledgement); the same basic emotions (angry, happy, scared, and sad); and the same basic abilities (rationality, logic, and communication). These are, of course, all human traits.

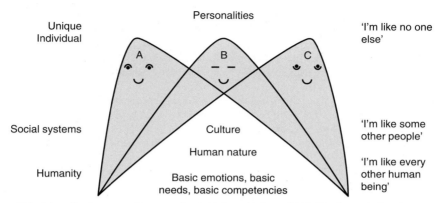

Figure 17.1 Intercultural conversation according to Hofman (Hofman, 2013). The figure depicts three people with elements which either correspond or don't. (Source: Interculturele gespreksvoering: theorie en praktijk van het TOPOI-model. Hofman. 2013. Bohn Stafleu van Loghum)

The second level indicates that the behaviour of these people is also determined by their social system and culture. These will differ to some extent (in language, knowledge, values/standards, symbols/rituals/heroes) and will be similar to some extent. Think of possible similarities in age, gender, education, musical interest, and so on. So besides a universal basis, the three differ from each other on points that are characteristic of the collective to which they belong. Interesting in this context is that research by Chugh *et al.* (1994) in Canada showed that health attitudes among different ethnic groups differed more within a cultural group than between different ethnic groups.

At the highest level in the model, personal contact takes place as the final form of communication. That level encompasses those unique physical and psychological attributes that make a person what they are: unique, like no other. These unique properties are partly innate and partly acquired. So intercultural communication is ultimately about personal contact: the contact between unique people, not between cultures.

Intercultural Communication: Attunement Is at the Centre of It All!

Intercultural communication is, above all, about interpersonal communication. This is communication between two people who are different, but also very similar at the same time. The communication between the two requires adjustment or attuning. Sometimes the attunement will take a little effort; other times it requires much more.

Now, what does this mean for your conversation? First of all, remember that there is a person in front of you who has the same basic needs as you (first level). Remember, too, that they partly talk/look/think differently to you and partly talk/think/look like you (second level). And finally, ensure that you see them as a unique person and make contact with them (third level). These three levels can help you to fulfil your role as a confidant and lay the foundation for your physiotherapy assistance and the other roles you fulfil.

A few specific hints:

- Think of the person as an individual and not as part of a 'culture'. So ask personal questions directed at the individual, not about their culture.
- Accurately observe non-verbal behaviour. For example, whether someone wants to shake your hand is often easy to see. If you have doubts about certain customs and whether or not they are appropriate, ask the patient. For example, 'I'm used to shaking hands with people. What do you prefer as a greeting?'

- At the start of the consultation, ask how to pronounce their name correctly and how the patient wants to be addressed. If a family member comes along, show your appreciation. Discuss whether an interpreter is desired, and if there is an interpreter, discuss their role during the consultation. Take different views on gender into account.
- When building on the relationship, be aware that non-verbal expressions are sometimes different to those you are used to.
- If you are in doubt about discussing certain topics, ask the patient if they want to talk about a certain topic. For example: 'Do you mind if I we discuss this further?' or 'How would you like it if we talk about this briefly?'
- If there are language barriers, be very careful to check that the patient understands your explanations.
- Keep in mind that shared decision-making is less common for some individuals (but probably still advisable).

Language Barrier

One complicating aspect in your conversation with the patient can be a language barrier. This can make it difficult to take up your role as a coach, communicative detective, and teacher in cases where this is crucial, and it inhibits bringing about a good relationship of trust. So how can you handle this as well as you possibly can?

Of course, using an interpreter can be part of the solution. But that's not always possible. In these instances, try to match your patient's language as closely as possible. If you notice that your patient uses sentences with five or six words and uses many of the same words repeatedly, adjust to this. Use the same words as the patient as much as possible and keep your sentences short. That may feel strange to you, but it makes your interaction a lot more effective.

Another consequence of your patient's insufficient language skills is that they will also have less knowledge about things that are often customary in your language and culture. For example, they know fewer nuances regarding pain experience and pain localisation or fewer nuances of the experience of tightness in COPD and are not able to put these nuances into words. You may have to do so with fewer distinctions than you're used to.

One last tip: many people have a tendency to speak with a raised voice when there is a language barrier. Of course that is not necessary, so watch out for this.

Health Literacy Skills

A bottleneck in intercultural communication often mentioned by physiotherapists is the assumptions made by foreign patients about the roles of the care worker and the patient in the recovery: namely, that the patient should have a passive role and the therapist has to solve it all. In fact, this view is probably not due to the cultural background of the patient. It is also seen among local patients, particularly among the elderly and those with less education. Most likely it has to do with reduced health literacy skills, (lack of) knowledge, and related attitudes. By talking to the patient about their knowledge and opinions regarding their health problem and your role as care worker, the patient may start to think differently about this. Be patient and understanding. In any case, it is not a good idea to simply 'go along' with the patient and give them a different (passive and less effective) treatment just because they seem to expect it. Your attunement is again crucial: match the patient's use of language and their level of knowledge. The guidelines you will find in Chapter 14 Section on health literacy skills, which are focused on low literacy, will also likely help here.

COMMUNICATING WITH CHILDREN

In communicating with children, you will perform the same core tasks during the consultations as with adults. In this respect, what is described in Parts I, II, and III of this book is no different.

What *is* different in communicating with children is how you approach the child and to what extent the child can bear responsibility. This depends on the child's level of cognitive, social, and emotional development. A child develops from complete dependency to independence and autonomy, while the parents are doing the opposite and withdraw increasingly as carers and educators as the child grows up. This is already difficult for many parents, but is certainly the case if they have a (chronically) ill child. This is something to take seriously and in which you can support the parents.

Children can participate in the discussion about their health and indicate their needs with regard to treatment from about the age of two (Nova *et al.*, 2005). From the age of six, children can participate (at least partially) in the decision-making concerning the treatment (Butz *et al.*, 2007). From about eight years of age, illness perceptions play a role and children are capable of a reasonable degree of self-management (Winkelstein *et al.*, 2000). From an early age, children can therefore be actively involved in the consultation (Stubbe, 2016).

The Role of Parents

The role of the parents in the health of the child is important—sometimes even more important than the child's own role. This is certainly the case with younger children. Parents then largely determine what the child does or does not do, due to the child's limited ability to take responsibility. This is why you want to be able to communicate effectively with both the child and the parents—and that is not easy in practice. If, during the first consultation, both the parents and the child are present, the conversation requires extra attention. For example, your verbal and non-verbal attunement with the parents will be different from that with the child. As a result, as a physiotherapist, you have to 'switch over' each time in order to achieve a balanced consultation in which you have sufficiently listened to and informed both the parents and the child.

Thinking laterally ■ **Talking to Two People**

There are many possible situations in which you, as a physiotherapist, may be in conversation with two or even more people: a child with their parent(s), an African woman who has brought along her child to interpret for her, an older man with his caregiver, and so on. For effective communication, this means that you have to develop a relationship with both of them. The partnership is no longer just between the patient and the physiotherapist—it becomes a team of three or four. Develop this extensive partnership carefully and don't just focus on the patient.

Hints for Communicating With Young Children

Entering into a relationship of trust with children up to 12 years of age requires extra attention (Stubbe, 2016). Young children are more likely to be afraid of a strange environment, and often naturally so. So you have to provide a suitable and pleasant child-friendly environment (think of toys, children's furniture, opportunities to entertain themselves, etc.). In addition, non-verbal behaviour and attunement play an important role. In fact, with an infant, this is the only form of communication you can use. This, of course, includes tactile contact. Posture, speaking tone, facial expressions, body language, and language use help to shape the role of confidant. As a child's cognitive development progresses, the content (that is, the verbal side) of communication becomes more important.

Involve the child in the consultation from the beginning. Do this immediately when you meet them—for example, by asking the child to introduce everybody. Ask the child whether they themselves want to say why they came or whether the parents should do this for them. One way to structure the conversation and allow the child to speak sufficiently is to agree at the beginning of the conversation that everybody should have a turn. When it is the child's turn, you ask them questions, explain things, and give the child the opportunity to ask their questions and tell their story. After some time, the parents then get their turn.

Gathering information while taking the history can be done not only in the traditional way, but also while playing with the child. For young children, use open questions and multiple choice questions, possibly adding questions which are more closed if the child finds it difficult to process more open dialogue. Using directive questioning is extremely useful because it allows you to indicate the topic you want to discuss while still asking an open question. For example, 'How do you feel about writing down some stuff?' or 'What do you find difficult about walking?' Encourage the child to express their emotions. Conduct the conversation with an enquiring and interested attitude; avoid intonation which indicates that something is right or wrong. In your communication, when you switch to the parents (or vice versa), you can do this effectively by first summarising what has been discussed up to that point.

The physical examination is initially performed on young children (up to about four years of age) while the child is sitting on the lap of one of the parents. Again, you often use games, images, and metaphors to help here. Be pragmatic: not everything can be examined as quickly as you would like. First choose things that make the child feel as comfortable as possible; as confidence grows, more can be done.

In the phase of 'explanation, decision-making, goal-setting, and planning' it is sometimes useful (especially in the case of young children) to ask the parent to explain this to the child. Then involve the child as much as possible in the decision-making process. Pictures, photos, and drawings help the child (and the parents) to remember things. In addition, give parents guidance for awkward situations at home: what to look out for and what to do in specific instances.

It is often useful to ask the parents if your communication with them and with the child went well. And you may ask if they have any suggestions to improve this. This way, you can optimally attune to them and the child.

Hints for Communicating With Older Children

In children (or teenagers) from about 12 years of age, aspects of interpersonal communication play a role related to brain development. A few points regarding the unique features of the developing adolescent's brain are worth keeping in mind:

- The capacity for abstract and hypothetical thinking is increasing. Because of this, an adolescent is able to understand the world better and they are more likely to approve or disapprove of something (in its entirety!). By making rational considerations, the young person is stimulated, and by matching these considerations with a good feeling or emotion, a strong motivation is created. If the adolescent is less capable of abstract thinking, discuss more concrete events and short-term consequences.
- The human stress response system matures, making it temporarily more sensitive. This is necessary in order to become independent, because in childhood, the parents protected the child and the function of this stress response system was less important. As a result, the young person can be more tense and sometimes more time is needed—you may have to invest more in the relationship and in mutual trust. In addition, the emotions of a young person are often stronger.
- The sleep–wake rhythm changes: young people become tired later in the evening than children, but have the same need for sleep. Because of this (and their ongoing physical development and growth), an adolescent regularly has less energy, and fatigue makes them more susceptible to stress. This may require extra patience on the part of the practitioner.

At the same time, the young person is developing a strong identity. They experiment and search for boundaries; the brain of an adolescent is enormously flexible and they want to make use of this flexibility. They investigate who they are and who they want to be, and they test and reflect this to others. Adolescents are more focused on peers and they separate themselves from their parents and other educators. What other young people think is therefore possibly more important than what you want to teach them. Resistance to your opinion may not be because of you or how you do things, but because of your role as a care worker and educator. Rejecting authority is really part of puberty, especially in an area that the adolescent themselves believe they know about. Keep in mind that if certain arguments do not suit the adolescent, they will try to find counter-arguments that are not always realistic.

Focal points for having a conversation with older children include:

- Make sure you have enough seating for everybody before you start the conversation.
- Focus primarily on the teenager and only in the second instance on the parents if they have come along. It is often desirable to do part of the consultation with the teenager alone.
- Don't always expect a structured story from a teenager.
- Attune to the person, their age, and their abilities: they're not too young, but also not too adult (overestimating them is easy). Watch your intonation! The role of confidant, for which equality is the basis, is essential with adolescents.
- Teenagers are sometimes shy and reserved. Take into account environmental factors that play a role and that you are not familiar with, such as the child's upbringing. The style of parenting makes quite a difference to how the child reacts to you. Is the child used to a warm or a cool approach? Are the parents dominant or lenient with the child? Give the teenager space and take your time. A young person needs more time to allow themselves to trust you and bond with you.
- Help them to express how they feel. Reflect on their feelings, and be open and curious to this.
- A teenager's emotions may be stronger and they often express them forcefully, but for all their intensity, they are not necessarily right. So don't be unnecessarily distracted by this.
- Ask open questions while gathering information and use some directive questioning if the teenager has difficulty answering.
- When doing a physical examination, it is good to ask the teenager who may be allowed at the examination. Start your examination with the part that causes the least discomfort.
- Involve the teenager as much as possible in decision-making while 'explaining, setting goals, and planning'. Give parents guidance for difficult situations ('action planning').

COMMUNICATION WITH THE ELDERLY

Communication with the elderly requires adaptation as soon as cognitive functions decline due to (physiological) changes in the older brain. This is noticeable in some at the age of 60, in others at the age of 85 ... or even later! For example, you might see a decrease in memory function and learning ability, in spatial orientation, and in the ability to think analytically, coupled with a decrease in language functions. This makes it difficult for the older patient to process a lot of information at the same time and to learn and remember many different new things one after the other. As a result, adapting to new situations and implementing new routines is more difficult. Moreover, it is often more difficult for the older person to gain and maintain insight into connections between certain things. When communicating with the elderly, you therefore primarily need to take into account the state of the 'older brain'. The extent to which you do this obviously depends on the extent to which that individual's brain functions have decreased. This is a very gradual process that is often difficult to estimate. In addition to these changes in cognitive functions, there are often auditory and visual problems (see Sections "Communication in the case of auditory impairment" and "Communication in the case of visual impairments").

In addition to physiological ageing, communication is often made more difficult by pathological changes seen in dementia. This process, too, is gradual and it is difficult to estimate what stage a person is in. That is why sensitivity is required for the extent to which you need to adjust your communication with the older person.

Finally, it is good to think about the phase of life in which the older person finds themselves. Being ill may have a different meaning for an older person now than when they were young. There may be increasing dependency, loneliness, or disabilities that may be permanent. What does this mean to them? A further issue is also what the patient expects from the physiotherapist, what they are used to, and whether (or how much) they want to be involved in the decision-making concerning the treatment. These aspects may require adjustment from you as a practitioner.

Guidelines for Communication With the Elderly

When communicating with an older patient, you quickly try to assess the extent to which you need to adapt your communication to 'the older brain'. This may require an active approach, because sometimes you won't notice anything different about an older person if you are letting them tell their own story. However, if you explicitly ask them about certain things and get an evasive answer or no answer at all, then you will need to pay closer attention. It is also sometimes wise to test whether what the patient says is correct, such as by asking if the patient can do things for you or by getting them to do something which they say they can do with you.

Effective communication with the elderly is achieved by attuning to as many aspects as possible (verbal, tempo, use of language, facial expressions, etc.), bearing in mind that the patient may be more dependent on routines and on the non-verbal component in communication due to age. This is because the verbal (cognitive) component becomes more difficult. Here are some general guidelines for effective communication (Herman & Williams, 2009).

- At the beginning of the conversation, carefully establish a relationship with the patient and their carer, paying attention to both. Let the carer participate in the conversation, ask them something once in a while. By specifically asking the carer something at regular intervals, you will prevent them from interfering all the time.
- Simplify your language and sentences. Use simple words that are as close as possible to the patient's own words, avoid jargon, and use short sentences with a simple structure in which the subject is at the beginning of the sentence. Limit yourself to one topic per sentence.
- Avoid condescending and derogatory language and tone.
- Often there are multiple health problems present. In this case, find out which problem deserves attention, in the patient's own estimation.
- Repeat regularly and give the patient an active role by having them repeat things themselves. Repeat in different ways (using slightly different words) and with different examples and objects. This allows you to stimulate other parts of their memory so that explanations can get through.
- When gathering information from them, older people can be verbose and spend a lot of time on irrelevant issues when talking about themselves. Look at what lies behind these irrelevant issues. Provide structure by summarising and encouraging further discussion of a specific topic by, for example, using directive questioning. Clarification of the request for help may require extra attention. Furthermore, embarrassment can play a role in certain themes; pay close attention to non-verbal signals.
- Moderate your pace and take your time, pause occasionally, spread the amount of information over a few consultations, and use metaphors less frequently.
- Write down important information point by point.
- Make more use of body language and body contact according to how cognitively approachable the patient is.
- In your therapy treatment, always approach the patient from their context and daily activities.

Guidelines for Communicating With Elderly People With Dementia

These guidelines apply to communication with all elderly people. However, it becomes more and more important as brain functions decline in the elderly. In the case of dementia, the following points are also important (Gillissen, 2014; Orange & Ryan, 2000; Williams, 2006):

- Don't talk *about* the patient but *with* them, even if communication becomes more difficult.
- In thinking and acting, accept the patient's reality and go along with them in your communication. Due to memory problems, the patient's reality is often different from ours. Accept this reality and do not enter into a discussion about whether something took place yesterday or last week or today.
- Beware of unnecessary and repeated 'testing' of the patient's memory. This makes them insecure and undermines your relationship of trust.
- Ask single questions, preferably closed questions (yes/no questions).
- Make emphatic use of non-verbal communication and provide clear and unambiguous signals, especially with regard to your facial expression. Also use touch to strengthen oral communication, get their attention, and make a connection.
- Make eye contact with the patient. This will help you keep their attention. Furthermore, eye contact can help to distract the patient from their emotional state if necessary, such as in the case of grief or anger.
- Excessively slow or loud talking is not necessary. Make sure you pause sufficiently in between your sentences.

COMMUNICATING WITH PEOPLE WITH INTELLECTUAL DISABILITIES

We speak of a moderate learning disability if someone has an IQ between 50 and 70. People with an IQ between 70 and 85 have a mild learning disability. In addition to someone's general IQ, social adaptability is of great importance in order to be able to speak of someone having a mild learning disability or difficulties. This section deals with communicating with people with moderate learning disabilities. Most aspects dealt with here also apply to communicating with people with mild learning disabilities. Earlier (in Chapter 14), the concept of health literacy was discussed. There's definitely an overlap here. A significant proportion of people with a mild learning disability also have impaired health literacy skills.

People with mild learning disabilities process information more slowly and often need more time to think about things. They are strongly focused on the present and on concrete matters and they often talk in short or stumbling sentences. Sometimes they use difficult words in the wrong way and/ or in the wrong context, or they pronounce them incorrectly. People with mild learning disabilities often do not understand the (full) consequences of their own actions and may find it difficult to scrutinise their own actions. They are often unable to recount exactly when something happened or was agreed upon. Emotions often have a major impact on them: they quickly become repetitive about emotional matters, even if they don't matter at the time. They don't always understand jokes and sometimes they take an expression that is meant figuratively, literally. Reading is often problematic, making written information less useful (American Psychiatric Association, 2013).

Of course, all of this has consequences for communication. The most important thing is that you are clear, concrete, and understandable. So use short sentences and simple words, and avoid using metaphors. Speak calmly and provide a quiet environment without distracting noises, and with a tidy and simple decor.

In addition, the following focal points apply:

- Give one assignment or message at a time.
- Listen carefully, ask questions, and regularly summarise (this gives structure and a base).
- Give the patient time; be patient.

- If there is something to choose from, limit the choice to two or three options.
- At the end of the conversation, check that your message has come across correctly.
- Search together for a way to properly schedule appointments. Ask: 'What's convenient for you?' or 'What shall we agree on?' Don't leave too much time in between appointments or the patient will forget about it.
- The lower the mental level of the patient, the more difficult language and words become. It is then advisable to work with well-considered and appropriate pictures, pictograms, and visual images.
- If you notice that these measures are not sufficient, find out if the patient can be accompanied by a parent, carer, or supervisor next time.
- Take into account a possible hearing impairment, which is more common in patients with a learning disability.
- Address the patient in a normal way about behaviour that causes annoyance or inconvenience. Give them tips on how to behave differently (Sullivan & Developmental Disabilities Primary Care Initiative Co-editors, 2011).

COMMUNICATION IN THE CASE OF AUDITORY IMPAIRMENT

About 6% of the world's population is hard of hearing or deaf. Due to hearing damage among young people and the ageing of the population, it expected that the number of people who have hearing impairments will only increase. The prevalence of hearing issues in the age group over 65 is about 30%. With an increase in age, this number increases (WHO, 2013).

Being slightly to profoundly hard of hearing means that a person can often still understand individual conversations (with or without the aid of a hearing aid and/or with voice elevation). Being severely hard of hearing to deaf means that it is not possible to have conversations without also using speech-reading or sign language.

The number of deaf people is considerably smaller than those who are hard of hearing, although the figures are mainly estimates (World Federation of the Deaf, 2020): probably about 70 million people in the world are severely hard of hearing or deaf, of which about half have prelingual deafness. The prelingual deaf were born deaf or became deaf before the third year of life. They usually have difficulty in language acquisition, which means that it is not only difficult to learn to speak, but also to acquire the language itself. And a language deficiency often leads to a knowledge deficiency. Deaf people therefore often have to make much more of an effort than hearing people to acquire knowledge and information. Generally, people who have only become deaf after learning to speak have fewer problems making themselves understood, as well as fewer problems with understanding language and acquiring knowledge and information.

Guidelines for Communication With Those Who are Slightly to Severely Hard of Hearing

- In the waiting room, try to make eye contact with the patient before you say their name.
- Speak calmly and articulate clearly. You may speak more loudly if the patient so desires. Avoid using subordinate clauses or roundabout approaches.
- Use facial expressions and natural gestures. Don't exaggerate.
- Keep eye contact: speak to the patient face to face.
- Don't hold anything in front of your mouth and make sure there is enough light so that your mouth is clearly visible. Don't stand with your back to the light.
- Reduce or eliminate background noise such as a radio or background music.
- Make sure to sit or stand close to the patient.
- Keep in mind that someone who is hard of hearing often first has to watch and/or listen to what you say before the content can penetrate. This can sometimes lead to a delayed reaction.

- The patient may not understand you right away. You might have to repeat what you said—if necessary, in different words.
- Occasionally ask the patient if they have understood everything correctly. In this way, you show understanding and make it easier for the patient to bring up any listening and/or comprehension problems.
- Write things down, such as parts of your explanation of the health problem, names, addresses, phone numbers, and dates of appointments. This avoids unnecessary misunderstandings (Commonwealth of Australia, 2009b; "Communicatietips", 2015a).

Hints for Communicating With the Deaf

Besides the tips given above for conversing with those who are hard of hearing, the following issues are important for communicating with deaf people who can lip read:
- Write down tricky words that are too difficult or impossible to guess.
- A deaf person cannot modulate the volume of their own voice to the ambient sound. Ask them to speak more loudly or softly if necessary.
- Let them pause every now and then. A deaf person can get tired of the conversation, such that they can no longer take in what is being said (Commonwealth of Australia, 2009b; "Communicatietips", 2015b).

To communicate with deaf people who cannot lip read, you may use the following tips:
- In the waiting room, try to make eye contact with the deaf patient before you say their name. Deaf people who cannot lip read can still often lip read their own name.
- You can draw their attention through body contact (e.g. by tapping on the shoulder). Do not approach the patient unnoticed from behind. They can't hear you coming and could take fright.
- Realise that for people who were born deaf, sign language is their first and natural language, and that to them spoken and written language is a second language—akin to French for a hearing English person. This means that they often don't learn to express themselves in English as fluently as hearing people, and that they may also have ongoing difficulty in spelling and reading English.
- Engage a sign language interpreter, or ask the patient to provide one (Commonwealth of Australia, 2009b).

COMMUNICATION IN THE CASE OF VISUAL IMPAIRMENTS

As a physiotherapist, you may also come into contact with the blind and visually impaired in your daily practice. The number of partially sighted people in the world is estimated at 217 million. In addition, about 36 million people are blind. Unfortunately, this number continues to increase (Flaxman *et al.*, 2017).

Communicating with a patient who is blind or partially sighted requires adjustment but isn't scary or complicated. By paying some attention, you can achieve a great deal.

Blind and partially sighted people need to orient themselves through other senses and take more time to determine where they are and where they need to go. If you want to help a blind or partially sighted person, always ask permission first.

The hardest thing for many care workers is the automatic way in which they assume that the patient can see things. For example, if you greet someone in passing, would a person who is blind know it is you? After all, they only hear 'good afternoon'.

Here are some suggestions for communicating with blind or partially sighted patients (Commonwealth of Australia, 2009a):
- Make sure the treatment room is tidy and easily accessible.
- Reduce or eliminate background noise such as a radio or background music.

- Set aside extra time for the consultation.
- When you collect the patient from the waiting room, ask them if they would like to put their hand on your shoulder so that they can follow you more easily.
- Assist them in entering the room and sitting down, if necessary.
- If a colleague or trainee attends the consultation, introduce them and ask permission as usual.
- At the start of the consultation, ask to what extent you need to take the visual impairment into account.
- The blind person has to rely fully on their hearing, so make sure you are well understood.
- When you explain things, do so in a well-structured and clear way. If you can use objects, they may be a suitable alternative to using pictures and illustrations. Place the objects or models you are using in the patient's hand so that they can feel them.
- If you write things down for the patient, it is usually more convenient to do so electronically, such as in an email, because most visually impaired people have software that reads out electronic text. Of course, it is also possible to record your explanation, for example with your phone or computer, and then send it by email.
- If you read out certain information or documents, such as the referral, refrain from reading out comments. If necessary, provide additional information afterwards.
- During the physical examination, make sure that you clearly indicate what you are doing, especially with hands-on tests, so that the patient is prepared for what is to come. If you are in doubt about being able to perform a certain test on the patient, consult them.
- Don't assume too quickly that something can't be done.

Summary

In this chapter, several groups of patients with whom you need to adapt your communication are discussed. These adaptations apply to all communication roles. At the same time, the manner in which the conversation is conducted does not differ substantially from the usual approach and the principles and working methods described in Parts I, II, and III apply.

When communicating with people from other (sub)cultures, the starting point is that people differ by their nature and that attunement is therefore central in the communication. Seeing the differences as logical and normal creates a good basis for conversation.

Communication with children is related to their cognitive and socio-emotional development. When communicating with younger children, you should ideally attune to the child's functioning level and speak to them about exactly that which they can talk about. Young people gradually develop the ability to think in an abstract way. This allows conversations to explore long-term consequences and goals which are further away.

A central focal point in communication with the elderly is the decline in cognitive functions. This makes it essential not to give too much information, to attune it to the needs of the patient, and to use tools to remember things well.

To communicate with the mentally disabled, taking their personal life experience into account is central: it must take place in the present. Using simple language focused on concrete matters is essential.

Adjustments in communication with people with auditory disabilities are not complicated. The action of looking (visus) plays a big role, and this should consistently be taken into account in communication. By giving priority to visual contact (eye contact, the ability to lip read) and only asking about or explaining things afterwards, this important condition is met.

In communicating with people with visual impairments, oral communication plays the most important role. First make contact by using speech, only using physical contact afterwards.

Finally, communication with these particular groups often involves a counsellor (parent or carer), which also requires an adjustment in your communication.

CHAPTER 18

Special Conversations and Forms of Conversation

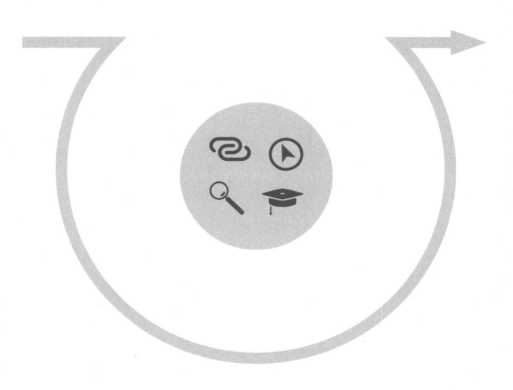

In the practice of physiotherapy, the conversation in the diagnostic process or the therapy process, as described in Chapters 3 to 11, is the most common conversation. Less common are the conversations in this chapter: conversations about loss or mourning, delivering bad news, and 'risk communication' (explaining specific health risks and data).

DEALING WITH LOSS AND MOURNING

Many clinicians may not be aware of it, but they probably come into regular contact with patients who are struggling with loss and mourning. Loss and mourning not only play a role when someone loses a loved one, but also when the patient is confronted with losing a job, loss of health, loss of status, and so on.

In the process of grief, a person performs a number of mourning tasks—activities that the mourning person can do to process their loss. These mourning tasks are (Keirse, 2011):

- accepting the reality of loss;
- processing the grief and pain;
- adjusting to the world (without the deceased, without health, without work);
- assigning a new place to the past (a new place for the deceased, a new place for the previous job/function, a new place for when they were healthy); and
- learning to love the present again.

As a physiotherapist, you can support the patient in this process from your role as a confidant. Your presence—being there for them—is the key (Keirse, 2011). You talk to the patient, listen to them, and support them emotionally. Knowledge about mourning tasks is useful in this respect, in order to better understand the patient, to have patience with them, and to approach them appropriately. Your role in dealing with the loss can even be important, without having to act as an expert. Only you can answer the question of whether you can and want to play a role in the patient's processing of grief. Guarding your professional role and your own boundaries is a focal point.

BREAKING BAD NEWS

In the practice of physiotherapy, you sometimes have to give the patient bad news, such as a certain analysis or diagnosis, or discontinuation of the treatment.

In most cases, you try to prevent this from being an unpleasant surprise by including the patient as much as possible in the diagnostic and therapeutic process, so that the patient can see for themselves what the (im)possibilities are and which way 'things are going'. This is discussed in Parts I, II, and III of this book. Unfortunately, this does not always work or is not possible in all cases.

To break bad news, you can use the step-by-step plan below (Silverman *et al.*, 2013; Staveren, 2010). Each step has a number of focal points. The plan forms a basis for your working method and is quite comprehensive in the physiotherapy context. You may want to omit certain steps, but that's up to you.

1. Preparation
   a) What should I tell the patient? Think carefully about what you want to say and write it down so that you can fall back on it during the conversation.
   b) Where should I tell them? Choose a suitable location and make a suitable arrangement.
   c) How should I tell them? For example, should family members be present, and how do you think the patient will react? Prepare for this.
2. Introduction
   a) Make contact with and attune to the patient. The basis for this conversation is your role as a confidant.

    b) **Introduction:** briefly tell them something about the purpose of the conversation and about how you want to conduct the conversation (in other words, set an agenda).

3. Breaking the bad news

    a) **Marking:** announce what you're about to say.

    b) **Chunking method:** give the bad news in simple short sentences, with the most important news first. Be honest and clear about what you want to say. In addition, remember that emotions greatly reduce the patient's ability to remember things and process complicated information, so watch out for information that is too overwhelming for the patient or too complicated.

4. Accepting the bad news

    a) **Show empathy:** empathise with the patient and their feelings and help them put this into words. Keep in touch, and make body contact if necessary, because that can sometimes say more than any remark. Listen to the patient and reflect what they say. Acknowledge and accept their emotion or lack of it at that moment.

    b) Help the patient deal with their emotions:

       i. **Grief:** if the patient becomes sad, identify the emotion with empathy and give it time and space. Don't be afraid of silence; on the contrary, it offers space for the patient's emotion.

       ii. **Anger:** sometimes patients get angry when hearing bad news, possibly also becoming angry with you as a therapist. Don't go on the defensive and don't respond unduly. Prioritise the emotion and the relationship between you and the patient by reflecting and attuning to the patient. Sometimes the anger seems to be directed at you, but in reality it is not.

       iii. **Confusion:** due to the impact the news has on the patient, they may be tempted to ask all kinds of questions, often fundamental or significant ones. Usually there is not much point in answering such questions directly, because the patient will hardly remember the answers at this time. Sometimes, however, it can be useful. It is often more useful to acknowledge the patient's needs and to discuss the source of their questions. In addition, reflections on the patient's feelings are appropriate.

5. Additional information

    a) Depending on how emotional the patient is, you now give additional information. If the emotions are still strong, you don't give much information because the patient will not process it.

    b) Make sure the patient understands everything. The best way to do this is to ask the patient to summarise the message in their own words and to ask further questions about the consequences of certain things.

    c) Find out what the patient still wants to know by asking them if they want to know more at this point and, if so, what.

    d) Check if the patient can remember this information and provide them with tools and background information.

6. Planning and support

    a) **Provide hope and perspective:** Be realistic about the perspective which you offer the patient. Support the patient by being positive where you can and letting them know that you will do as much as you can to work with them on improvement.

    b) **Come to a shared decision:** After discussing the physiotherapy analysis, a shared decision about the treatment approach often follows. It may be a good idea to only discuss the treatment options generally and to make a follow-up appointment to come to a decision.

7. Conclusion

    a) Conclude the conversation by going over what you discussed together. You will also make appointments for the future.

The hardest steps in this conversation are step 3 (giving the bad news) and 4 (accepting the bad news). Many have a tendency to soften the blow by, for example, using diminutives (when this is not appropriate), avoiding certain words, and proposing solutions too quickly. However, make sure that you complete step 3 so that it is clear what is going on, and only then move on to step 4 to help with the processing of the message. By asking the patient how it has affected them, you give them room to express their emotions.

The conversation in which you give bad news can be a stressful situation for you as a physiotherapist (Ptacek *et al.*, 2001; Saraiya *et al.*, 2010). Good preparation and following the step-by-step plan mentioned here can reduce this to some extent. Keep in mind that, in the end, patients want you to be honest with them and tell them what's really going on (Heyland *et al.*, 2009).

RISK COMMUNICATION

Sometimes physiotherapists use specific data such as figures from scientific research in their explanations or education provision. This is called 'risk communication', an activity appropriate to the task and role of a teacher or a communicative detective. Scientific data is often difficult for patients to understand. This is partly due to the way in which the data is explained to the patient. If, for example, someone says that 'this doubles the chance of recovery', at first this seems great. But the chance of recovery here is a 'relative risk'. In other words: in this case, this could mean that the chance of recovery was initially 2%, doubling to 4%. Seen in absolute terms, this remains only a small chance for recovery. In short, this is not a useful way to explain figures to patients.

Here are some focal points for a more effective approach (Epstein *et al.*, 2004; Fischhoff, 2012):

- Name frequencies of occurrence and not the probability of single events, such as by saying: 'Of every 10 patients who have this problem, three recover without help and seven with help'.
- Name natural frequencies (and not conditional probabilities) by saying: 'Every year, five out of 1,000 people get a herniated disk of the lower back. It is known that out of 100 people with a herniated disc, 75 recover without surgery'. (These numbers are just an example.)
- Name the absolute risks and not the relative risks. Say, for example: 'Of the 100 people being operated on for a herniated disk, 21 recover well within two years. With 79 people, residual complaints remain'. (The numbers are just an example.)
- Always use fixed denominators: 10, 100, 1,000, and so on, not 30 or 200 or 600, etc. Keep using that denominator and change it only when really necessary.

The disadvantage of numbers is often that they are only numbers. Patients can't always see what you want to say with the numbers. However, there are various ways to make a number meaningful to the patient. You can keep in mind the following tips:

- Give the figures a different perspective by comparing them with something the patient can picture for themselves. For example: 'If opened out into a continuous sheet, the area of all lung vesicles is 70 to 100 square meters. That's as big as the training room you just saw. Because of your illness, you can actually use only half of your lung vesicles. So you have to do everything with an area as large as half the training hall. That means you are getting considerably less air'.
- Use a risk ladder. With this, you are relating the chance of a certain event to the behaviour and characteristics of the patient. In Figure 18.1, the risk of developing type 2 diabetes is related to weight and exercise behaviour. This also gives the possibility, as in this example, of relating a certain risk to multiple causes and it gives the patient the possibility to choose which cause they want to tackle first.
- Make the figures visual by using a frequency drawing, graph, or table (Figures 18.2a–c). Think of bar graphs, pie charts, and frequency tables with icons.

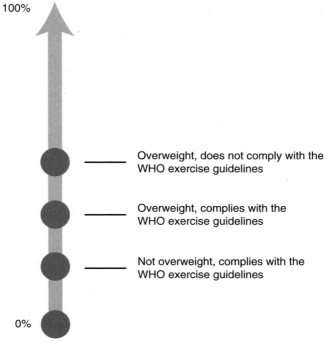

Overweight, does not comply with the WHO exercise guidelines

Overweight, complies with the WHO exercise guidelines

Not overweight, complies with the WHO exercise guidelines

Figure 18.1 An example of a risk ladder.

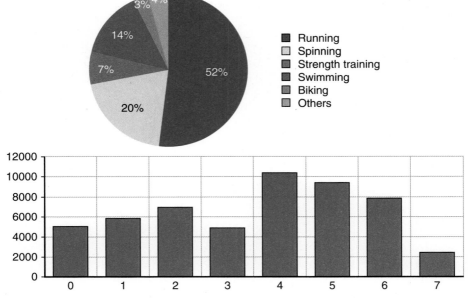

Figure 18.2 Examples of (a) pie chart, (b) bar graph, and (c) frequency chart.

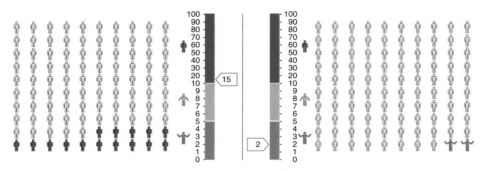

Figure 18.2   Cont'd

Summary

In this chapter, a few specific conversations are discussed, such as conversations about loss or mourning, breaking bad news, and risk communication.

In conversation with patients mourning the loss of a loved one, of a job, or of their health, your presence is central. As a physiotherapist, you try to support the other person in fulfilling their mourning tasks from your role as a confidant, insofar as you see this as appropriate and necessary for a professional.

Giving bad news, such as the discontinuation of treatment when the patient (and/or their parents/carers) may still see it as meaningful, can be a stressful situation. It requires preparation, followed by a calmly communicated and clear message, after which you help the patient to cope with the bad news.

The use of specific data relating to risks and chances of recovery is called risk communication. By mentioning natural frequencies and absolute risks, possibly while using graphs and frequency tables, you give the patient a realistic picture of their chances and risks.

CHAPTER 19

Talking About Stress and Lifestyle

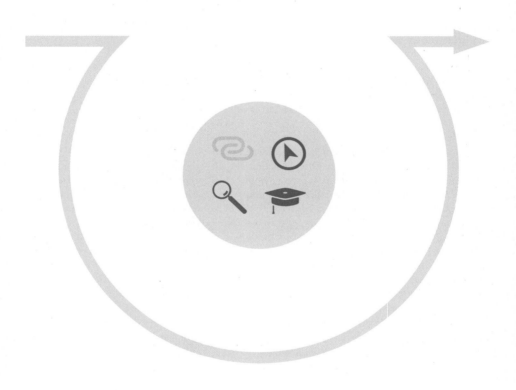

Discussing themes such as stress and lifestyle with the patient is sometimes seen as 'difficult'. At the same time, these factors are often very relevant because they reveal a cause of the health problem or a prognostically adverse factor. With a good analysis and, where possible, a suitable solution for these issues, you offer a more 'complete' form of assistance.

MAKING A CONNECTION BETWEEN THE HEALTH PROBLEM AND STRESS

Stress plays a role in a significant proportion of musculoskeletal syndromes in which pain is the most important symptom (Mallen *et al.*, 2007; Ramond-Roquin *et al.*, 2015). Stress, then, is a causal factor or an obstacle to recovery (Østerås *et al.*, 2015). In this respect, think of lower back pain (Grotle *et al.*, 2005; Parreira *et al.*, 2018), neck pain (Linton, 2000), and headaches (Boardman *et al.*, 2005). For example, 30% of patients who visit a primary care physiotherapy practice in the Netherlands have moderately to strongly increased stress scores (Horst *et al.*, 2005).

Some background knowledge about stress is important in order to have an adequate discussion with the patient about the connection between their health problem and stress. That is why this section will first address this issue, albeit briefly. More background information can be found in publications by Cooper and Folkman (Cooper & Quick, 2017; Folkman, 2011). This is followed by a conversation with the patient in which stress will be discussed.

Stress

Stress literally means 'tension', and is caused by a stressor. A stressor is the condition, situation, or event that causes the stress. One's reaction to the stressor is the stress response: the psychophysiological process that is expressed in physical, cognitive, emotional, and behavioural terms. The word 'stress' therefore refers to the process that is a consequence of the stressor and at the same time gives rise to the stress response. In the literature, the term 'distress' is often used to indicate an 'overload state' and carries negative associated emotions. The counterpart to distress is 'eustress', stress which has a positive connotation.

Distress is an emotional reaction to a situation (stressor). This emotional reaction of the patient arises from their perception of the situation in which they find themselves. This does not have to be an actual situation, but can primarily or even entirely take place in the patient's own thoughts or emotions. The thought of a threat can cause as much stress as an actual threat! The essential point is that with distress, the person wants to have control of the situation, but doesn't. The emotional reaction to distress can be reduced to three of the four 'basic emotions': angry, scared, sad, happy. When we're stressed, we feel angry, scared, or sad. The patient's emotions are often a combination of two of these basic emotions. For example, 'frustration' is a combination of anger and sadness (grief). Because this emotional reaction can be volatile (for example, in a repetitive but short-lived situation at work or at home), the emotion is not always recognisable to the patient and the stress response can also be limited, such that the patient does not immediately recognise the distress as being relevant to their health problem.

Different Stressors

Stressors can be classified in the following way.
- **Everyday concerns:** These are the relatively small daily events or situations that a person may have to deal with and which, when 'added together', can ultimately be experienced as burdensome by the individual. Such daily worries can therefore become a stressor. Think also of situations that briefly elicit stress (such as saying something at a meeting) and to which the person cannot accustom or adapt themselves to, such that the situation continues to elicit stress. For most people, a number of everyday situations may provoke a stress response, such as (prolonged) noise, a busy environment when they need to concentrate, lack of sleep, certain drugs such as alcohol, and being in a situation where they feel too hot. Work pressure is frequently mentioned as well (Lazarus, 1986; Schaufeli, 2006).

- **Life events:** These are major emotional events in a human life, whether positive or negative. Examples include: death of a loved one, losing a job, getting married, having a child, changing jobs, or having a seriously ill partner. Known in this context are the life events as listed by Holmes and Rahe (1967). They researched the connection between life events, distress, and the onset of disease. Eventually, they put together a ranking of stressful life events. This research and ranking have been much criticised. Nevertheless, the list may be useful as a concretisation of possible life events that contribute to experiences of stress.
- **Prolonged positive stress:** Prolonged positive stress and too few possibilities for recovery can eventually lead to distress. The fatigue that slowly builds up because the patient asks a lot of themselves activates the stress system; a prolonged neurohormonal activation ('arousal') takes place which can eventually exhaust the inhibitory and selective systems (Van Houdenhove, 2005).
- **Underloading:** Underloading is also increasingly described as a cause of distress. In contrast to prolonged and exhausting distress which can lead to burnout, we now also talk of a 'boreout'. The stressors here are boredom and lack of challenge and purpose (O'Brien, 2019).
- **Slow 'unwinding':** This is the case when the stress system remains active after a stressful situation and only returns to its basic level of activity very slowly. The neurohormonal reactions, of which the stress response is the expression, always take some time to 'extinguish'. With slow unwinding, this process is slower than normal. The cause may be that the stress system is not curbed properly by the inhibiting systems or that, although the stressful situation is over, the patient's emotions do not return to normal levels (van Houdenhove, 2005).
- **The patient's state of health:** This is a special situation in which the patient's own state of health now puts them under stress. In other words, the patient is anxious or worried about their health or their health problem so that it becomes a source of distress and a stress response arises (Folkman, 2011).

The Stress Response

Distress can be partially recognised by the stress response. This psychophysiological reaction is expressed in four dimensions: behavioural, cognitive, emotional, and physical. Within these four dimensions, numerous phenomena that are characteristic of the stress response are described, especially as they become more frequent (Compernolle, 1999). Behavioural responses include agitation, carelessness, apathy, arguing more often, or being less productive. Cognitive reactions include an increase in forgetfulness and confusion, brooding, or increased indecisiveness. Examples of emotional reactions include an increase in anxiety, uncertainty, and gloominess and/ or a decrease in calmness and sexual interest. In a physical sense, stress is characterised by insomnia, fatigue, restless movements, sweating, digestive problems, heart palpitations, and so on. A more complete overview of the symptoms of the stress response within the four dimensions can be found on Evolve.

Clinically, it is sometimes difficult to determine whether there are symptoms which are characteristic of a stress response or not. The reason for this is that many symptoms are volatile and that the patient may not be aware of all the symptoms.

Not every stress response is equally threatening to 'someone's health. The duration of the distress in particular determines whether this is the case: the longer the distress persists, the more the threat to health generally increases. Stress can also lead to other disorders and problems, such as depression, anxiety, and overexertion.

Assessing Distress

When discussing the theme of distress with the patient, it is first of all important to normalise this theme—that is, discuss it as much as possible as a normal theme, the same as you do with other themes and topics that you give a place to during a consultation. Considering distress as a special and/or tricky topic may in fact lead to unnecessary caution, which in itself will cause discomfort in your contact with the patient.

If you need a systematic approach to assess distress as a causal or restorative factor, you can use the following step-by-step plan (Hagenaars & Bos, 2010). Each of the following steps will make your notes a little more incisive. Depending on your goal and your competencies, you can abandon taking notes after each step (and possibly resume doing so at a later date). The step-by-step plan allows you to make a list and a partial analysis in relation to the distress. Notably, by adhering to the system described here, you are less likely to become involved in the patient's private life.

The steps below describe the question underlying your conversation with the patient: *What* do you want to investigate? You will find helpful questions in the Question Lexicon (available on Evolve) which will help you to know *how* to conduct the conversation.

- **Step 1:** Does the patient understand that there may be a connection between health problems in general and distress?
- **Step 2:** Does the patient understand that there may be a connection between their current health problem and distress?
- **Step 3:** Does the patient feel that there is a connection between their current health problem and distress?
- **Step 4:** Do they experience symptoms (physical, behavioural, cognitive, emotional) of the stress response?
- **Step 5:** Which stressor plays a causal role, your own state of health or something else? If it is the latter, are these everyday concerns, life events, prolonged positive stress, underloading, or slow unwinding?
- **Step 6:** What emotion is involved in relation to the named stressor?

Now for a brief explanation of these steps. First: the step-by-step plan forms a system that you can use as a therapist. As indicated above, it is not necessary to literally ask the patient the questions mentioned; they are intended as a guideline for the structure of your conversation. If you notice that the patient has insufficient knowledge (e.g. in steps 1 or 2) try to give them the right information first. Make sure your explanation is not too extensive and give concrete figures if these are known. Find out more about how to effectively communicate data in the Section "Risk communication" of Chapter 18.

In steps 1 and 2, start with a question each time in order to find out what knowledge the patient has of the issue. You might ask: 'What do you know about the connection between tension and health?' Furthermore, paying attention to the construction in the first three steps is important to leave the patient open to discussing stress as part of their health problem. It can also help if you ask the patient's permission to discuss the subject of distress with them. If you go too fast in the initial phase and do not include the patient sufficiently in your analysis, a misunderstanding or even dissonance may arise between the patient and yourself, making it less possible to discuss the subject.

In the fourth step, you record the presence or absence of phenomena in the behavioural, cognitive, emotional, and physical dimensions. If there are numerous expressions of the stress response, these notes will often lead to an insight into the highly probable presence of distress in the patient. If the patient comes to this insight, you can take the fifth step and look for the stressor. First you try to distinguish between distress caused by the health problem itself and distress caused by a situation or event outside the health problem. This is important because it affects the therapy plan; this will be discussed more in the next section.

In the sixth and last step, you help the patient to express which emotion is connected to the stressor. If the patient has difficulty putting this into words, you can use the basic emotions: angry, scared, sad, and happy. Say, for example: 'It might help you to put into words how you feel about yourself—what the situation is doing to you. I often use those emotions which are most common in people, namely: angry, scared, and sad. Which one of these three comes closest to how you feel in that stressful situation?' Or say: 'If you were to express your feelings in relation to this situation, would you be angry, sad, or scared?'

Conducting the Discussion on Dealing With Stress

If after a good review and analysis, it appears that stress plays a role in the patient's health problem, the question is: What now?

At the very least, part of your approach will aim to give the patient a deeper insight into the connection between stress and their health problem. Education provision aimed at a better understanding of illness with regard to the role of stress therefore always plays a part in addressing this situation.

Education provision on the connection between stress and the health problem includes a number of themes:

- acute and chronic stress;
- the neural component and the hormonal component of stress;
- the effects of acute and chronic stress;
- the specific connection to the patient's health problem.

The depth and comprehensiveness with which you address these themes in education provision will vary, and depend on:

- the information the patient needs to gain insight;
- the place that stress occupies in the patient's health problem; if stress occupies an important place as a cause and/or part of the health problem, learning about it will be considerably more extensive and in-depth than if it is only a relevant but minor factor in the recovery and/or occurrence.

Learning about the phenomenon improves the patient's understanding of the connection between their health problem and stress. Possible consequences also become clear, such as the chance of a slower recovery or a recurrence of the complaints. This insight enables the patient, together with the physiotherapist, to determine how important it is to improve their stress management. A small part of this could be tackled together with the physiotherapist, such as learning relaxation techniques aimed at reducing the stress response.

The importance that the patient attaches to stress in relation to their health problem will partly determine what they want to do with the stressful situation: wait, address, or accept. Although addressing the source of stress is of course the ideal situation, it does not always succeed. With this aspect, it is also helpful to realise that as a physiotherapist, you only play the role of confidant and discussion partner, not that of an expert.

The physiotherapist, as an expert, can however do something for the patient with regard to the stressor in some cases. If the stressor is formed by the patient's own health problem, then an explanation of it (what is going on, where does it come from, how can you recover from it) may possibly reduce the stressor, in turn reducing the stress response.

MAKING A CONNECTION BETWEEN THE HEALTH PROBLEM AND LIFESTYLE

An unhealthy lifestyle is probably the most important illness-causing factor in Western civilisation (Bodai *et al.*, 2018). Too little exercise, eating unhealthily and too much, smoking and drinking too much alcohol—these all threaten people's health. In this context, many patients who visit a physiotherapist have a health problem that is related to their lifestyle. Sometimes the lifestyle is causative, while in other cases the lifestyle acts as an inhibiting factor in the patient's recovery. Such cases include patients with back pain (Heneweer, 2011), neck pain, vascular disease (heavy smokers are 2.7 times more likely to have intermittent claudication) (Hirsch *et al.*, 2006), and COPD (smoking is almost always the cause of COPD) (Doll *et al.*, 2004).

Physiotherapists are often inclined to neglect asking about lifestyle while taking the (medical) history or may only ask if the patient exercises enough, which is just one of the aspects of lifestyle. This is unfortunate because it means that the health problem is not fully analysed; possible recovery or causal factors remain and/or the patient may not be (sufficiently) aware of the relationship between their health problem and their lifestyle.

When the concept of lifestyle is discussed in healthcare, the factors of exercise, smoking, alcohol, nutrition, and relaxation (rest) are frequently mentioned. If the patient's health problem may be caused by their lifestyle, then as a physiotherapist, you should make an attempt to examine that patient's lifestyle. You can then provide the patient with insight into the cause of their health problem and/or possible obstacles to recovery. This makes it possible to discuss with the patient whether they want to do something about their lifestyle, and if so, how they can do this and whether they need help from a (different) professional.

Put Into Action: Making a Connection Between the Health Problem and Lifestyle

Assessing lifestyle factors is very similar to assessing stress, and you do it on the basis of normalising the theme. To do so, you ask directly and in a normal way about the possible connection between the patient's health problem and their lifestyle.

If you need a systematic approach, the following step-by-step plan may help you.

- **Step 1:** Does the patient understand that there *may* be a connection between their current health problem and their lifestyle (exercise, smoking, alcohol, nutrition, relaxation)?
- **Step 2:** Does the patient feel that there *is* a connection between their health problem and their lifestyle?

First, ask the patient's permission to discuss their lifestyle. Next, in steps 1 and 2, you try to start with a question each time. For example, ask at step 1: 'Are you aware that your health is affected by habits such as too little exercise, smoking, too much alcohol, unhealthy eating, and insufficient rest?' Then continue with step 2: 'How do you see the connection between your lifestyle and your current complaints?' Or ask: 'To what extent do you think your current complaints are related to your lifestyle?'

If the patient indicates that they are unaware of the connection between lifestyle and health, you can ask if you may tell them a thing or two about this. You then give the patient brief and concise information. If necessary, give concrete figures (see the Section "Risk communication" in Chapter 18). The insight you give the patient into their health problem in relation to their lifestyle and the importance of this makes the lifestyle theme more relevant to the patient, and therefore more likely to be up for further discussion. Then, together with the patient, you can go through the five lifestyle aspects and make an assessment of how matters stand.

Some points of interest regarding lifestyle elements include the following:

- Expertise is required to make an incisive assessment of lifestyle factors, such as smoking, alcohol consumption, and nutrition. It is therefore a good idea to do an initial orientation and leave any follow-up to other care providers (dietician, general practitioner, psychologist).
- It is a human tendency to judge one's own behaviour more positively than it actually is. People 'gloss over' their unhealthy habits to themselves and thus to the outside world. Think of a smoker who maintains that they smoke 'with a filter' or 'only a few cigarettes a day', or someone who 'only' drinks two glasses of alcohol a day but who can't make an exception to this rule. Keep this in mind.
- When it comes to exercise, too, many people judge their own exercise behaviour more positively than it actually is. By being specific (asking questions and giving examples),

you weaken this effect. Using a 'pedometer, smartwatch, or fitness tracker' can also help by providing evidence of actual patterns.

- Nutrition is a difficult and comprehensive factor to analyse. A logical first step is to ask the patient about their weight and height and then calculate the BMI. This gives an indirect indication of their diet. A second step can be a global assessment of the dietary pattern based on the recommendations of the British Nutrition Foundation. Further analysis should be left to an expert.
- Relaxation (and rest) is included in an assessment of the presence of stress (see the previous section), the interchange between work and rest, and both the quality and quantity of sleep.

Put Into Action: A Conversation About Lifestyle Change

If the final conclusion is that lifestyle factors play a role in the patient's health problem, the next step is to provide education. If necessary, explain the connection between the patient's health problem and one or more lifestyle factors. This can help the patient to consider whether they want to do something about their lifestyle. As a physiotherapist, you may be able to act as the patient's coach in this area. The patient ultimately decides whether they want to tackle an aspect of their lifestyle and what support they want (and from whom) in doing so. Ambivalence and the self-efficacy of the patient also often play a role in changing their lifestyle. Addressing this is useful in order to increase the patient's motivation for a healthier lifestyle.

As a physiotherapist, you may also have a role as a coach/therapist when it comes to exercise. Keep in mind that mentoring a lifestyle change is a great challenge that requires the necessary expertise. This book does not deal with this any further.

Summary

In this last chapter of Part IV, the conversation with the patient about the connection between their health problem and stress and/or their lifestyle is discussed. By treating this conversation as normal—that is, as a normal theme of the physiotherapy conversation—this goes smoothly in most cases. Additionally, a simple step-by-step plan is provided for stress and lifestyle, which can form a guideline for the discussion about these topics.

PART V

Scientific Research

In 1998, Jonathan Silverman published his now famous book *Skills for Communicating with Patients* (Silverman *et al.*, 1998), in which the communication between the doctor and the patient was developed on the basis of scientific knowledge. The investigations described by Silverman opened the eyes of many care workers: communication mattered! Silverman's painstaking work towards the publication of his book would be considerably easier to do nowadays: a lot of information is more accessible. But above all, there is much more scientific research available on communication with patients. The fifth part of this book gives a selection from this research.

The four roles—confidant, coach, communicative detective, and teacher—have been retained as a structure to organise the large number of scholarly publications cited. A separate chapter is dedicated to each role. In addition, the chapters contain suggestions for the reader who is looking for more scientific research and background. The titles of the various subsections are based on the keywords commonly used in scientific research and literature.

The physiotherapy consultation

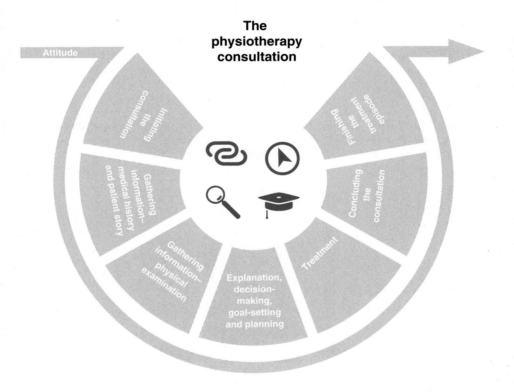

CHAPTER 20

The Role of Confidant

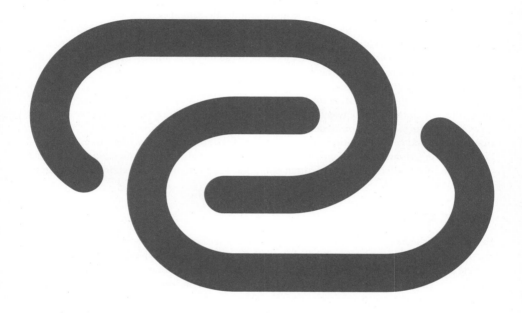

The confidant is a role that does not need professional expertise, but has as its foundation the interpersonal connection. This is often referred to as the therapeutic alliance. Also widely used is the concept of common factors, rather than those specific factors which partly determine the treatment effect. In addition, research into placebo effects provides interesting insights into the importance of the role of confidant. Despite the fact that these concepts overlap considerably, they have been described separately in the following paragraphs for the sake of clarity.

A section at the end concerns the physiotherapist's use of words.

Before discussing a selection of the scientific research into the above concepts, we can first lay a foundation. A systematic review by Carla Bastemeijer (Bastemeijer *et al.*, 2016) has described what patients crave in the sort of help they receive from healthcare practitioners. Seven values emerged as the most prized: uniqueness, autonomy, compassion, professionalism, responsiveness, partnership, and empowerment. To put it more simply: the patient needs to be seen as a person and an individual; to have freedom of choice; to have the care worker show involvement, professionalism, and responsibility, and encourage the patient and trust in their potential; and to have the patient and care worker work with each other. In the help you offer as a physiotherapist, the patient must therefore recognise these values as a basic attitude.

Mary O'Keefe and colleagues (2016) carried out a systematic review and meta-analysis in which they investigated what, according to the view held by patients and physiotherapists, determines the interaction between the patient and the physiotherapist in a positive sense. It gives concrete form to what Bastemeijer's study describes. Therapists should have the following interpersonal and communication skills: active listening, empathy, being friendly, encouraging and motivating, showing confidence in the patient, non-verbal attuning, and making (physical) contact. According to Nicole Brun-Cottan *et al.*, this is the 'art' of physiotherapy (Brun-Cottan *et al.*, 2018).

THE RELATIONSHIP

In a review of the literature, Mauksch concluded that the relationship between the care worker and the patient is of great importance for efficient dialogue in the consultation room. He mentioned in particular that setting the agenda jointly with the patient, noticing emotional and social signals, and building up and maintaining the rapport make the consultation more efficient (Mauksch *et al.*, 2008). In-depth listening to what the patient has to say, showing interest/questioning, and noticing and responding to the patient's concerns and emotions are important for a good cooperative relationship with the patient, the 'therapeutic alliance' (Pinto *et al.*, 2012; Testa & Rossettini, 2016).

This 'therapeutic alliance' often predicts (part of) the treatment result, as several studies have shown (Brunner *et al.*, 2019; Ferreira *et al.*, 2013; Schönberger *et al.*, 2006), such as in patients with pain or with an acquired brain injury.

So a better relationship gives better treatment results. A good treatment relationship can also enhance the patient's self-efficacy (Burns & Evon, 2007; Maisto *et al.*, 2015).

COMMON FACTORS

In 2010, Hall *et al.* (Hall *et al.*, 2010) conducted a systematic review of the role of the 'common factors' in the physiotherapy treatment of patients with a brain injury, musculoskeletal pain, heart failure, or multiple diseases. These non-specific factors, which mainly include the relationship and contact between the therapist and the patient, have an effect on the treatment result, according to Hall's review. The results of the various studies included were unfortunately difficult to 'pool'. Hall concluded that common factors have a positive correlation with (1) therapy compliance in patients with a brain injury and patients with multiple pathologies; (2) depressive symptoms in patients with heart failure and a brain injury; (3) treatment satisfaction in patients with musculoskeletal conditions; and (4) physical functioning in geriatric patients and patients with lower back pain.

Studies on 'compassionate care' also powerfully demonstrate the benefits of the relationship between patient and therapist, warm and kind-hearted treatment, and the promotion of autonomy. Several results show an improvement, as Stephan Post describes in an interesting review. Think about wound healing, therapy compliance, and general well-being (Post, 2011). The incidental discovery is just as interesting! The care worker suffers less burnout, fewer depressive symptoms, and is more likely to feel that their work 'really matters'.

PLACEBO EFFECTS AND COMMUNICATION

The work of Josien Bensing, professor of clinical and health psychology at Utrecht University in the Netherlands, has become nationally and internationally renowned because of her research and publications on the power of communication in generating and enhancing the placebo effect. There is healing power in the relationship which the care worker enters into with their patient, she argues. Paying attention, making contact, empathic listening and reflecting what the patient means, and picking up emotional signals are abilities that are part of this effect. An empathic basic attitude helps the patient to tell their story and makes them more involved (Derksen et al., 2013). This basic attitude characterises the role of confidant. Some interesting studies by Bensing are:

- Fassaert, T., Dulmen, S. van, Schellevis, F., Jagt, L. van der, Bensing, J. (2008) Raising positive expectations helps patients with minor ailments: A cross-sectional study. *BMC Family Practice, 9,* 38.
- Bensing, J. M., Verheul, W., van Dulmen, A. M. (2008) Patient anxiety in the medical encounter: A study of verbal and nonverbal communication in general practice. *Health Education, 108,* 5, 373–383.
- Bensing, J. M., Verheul, W. (2010) The silent healer: The role of communication in placebo effects. *Patient Education and Counseling, 80,* 3, 293–299.

That the placebo effect has an extremely strong effect has been demonstrated by the research of Raine Sihvonen, published in *The New England Journal of Medicine* (Sihvonen et al., 2013). In this study, 142 patients with a degenerative meniscus tear of the knee were divided into two groups. The study was multicentre, randomised, and double-blind. One group actually underwent an arthroscopic procedure in which a partial meniscectomy was performed. The other group was given a simulated arthroscopic procedure in which the meniscus was not operated on. The results were the same for both groups, measured with the Lysholm score, WOMET, and pain.

Placebo effects can also be evoked through the role of the confidant by being empathic, building a good working relationship with the patient, and being positive about the expected recovery. It is important to influence the patient in a positive direction by using certain words (with a positive connotation) and avoiding other words (with a negative connotation). Compare 'this is a good exercise' with 'this can be a good exercise'. The work of Frabizio Benedetti and Andrea Evers should not go unmentioned in the context of these placebo effects and communication. Benedetti and Evers showed neuropsychological and psychobiological changes that ultimately led to better treatment outcomes (Benedetti et al., 2013, 2016a, 2016b; Evers et al., 2014, 2018).

VOCABULARY AND NOCEBO

A number of studies show that the physiotherapist's use of words matters (Lown, 1996). The research of Heritage, for example, is interesting (Heritage et al., 2007). She found that patients reacted better (that is, more often) to the question: 'Is there anything else you wanted to bring up in this conversation?', than to the question: 'Are there any further issues you wanted to raise?' This may be because the second question somewhat evokes the idea that there 'shouldn't be any further issues'. Small nuances in word usage make a big difference.

Researchers have used fMRI scans to investigate what happens in the brain when words with a certain 'connotation' are used for pain. They came to the conclusion that words used during painful medical procedures affect the degree of pain and discomfort the patient experiences during the procedure. Words that are related to pain can activate the pain neuromatrix. Patients report more pain and discomfort if the explanation of the procedure is about how painful it is and if the procedure is explained using words related to pain (Ritter *et al.*, 2019).

Another interesting study is Darlow's. He interviewed people with acute and chronic lower back pain (Darlow *et al.*, 2013). His findings were that explanations previously given to patients sometimes have very unfavourable effects on these patients' illness perceptions, particularly when professionals refer to instability, weakness, adjusting or correcting the back, not bending down, to be careful, to avoid stress, and so on. What was particularly striking was the disastrous effect of the explanation, which gave patients the idea that their backs needed protection and were vulnerable. Although well-intentioned, explanations such as these therefore have an undesirable effect: the patient's illness perceptions become more negative and the prognosis deteriorates.

So being careful with your own language is advisable (Cuyul-Vásquez *et al.*, 2019)! The scientific research is clear about this (Benedetti, 2002; Evers *et al.*, 2018; Heritage *et al.*, 2007; Malani, 2010; Peper *et al.*, 2013; Ritter *et al.*, 2019; Testa & Rossettini, 2016; van Laarhoven *et al.*, 2011).

Finally, a publication which should not go unmentioned here is *Prioritising Person-Centred Care. Enhancing Experience* by National Voices (*Prioritising person-centred care. Enhancing experience*, 2014). This is a report giving a total of 110 studies on the patient experience and suggestions to improve it. It deals with a style of communication that focuses on understanding and cooperation, involving patients in decision-making, and providing good information to patients.

CHAPTER 21

The Role of Coach

The role of coach is aimed at strengthening the patient's autonomous motivation and supporting behavioural change. The targets for change are achieved from the patient's point of view. Therapy compliance is, of course, also a task of the coach. In this chapter, you will learn more about the scientific backgrounds of all these aspects.

MOTIVATIONAL INTERVIEWING

The role of coach is basically aimed at strengthening the patient's autonomous motivation. You're guiding the patient towards healthy behaviour. If you do this, it is important to communicate in such a way that the patient experiences a sense of freedom of choice and free will. The counterpart of this (and not part of the role of coach) is to put pressure on people by forcing them to take part in the conversation. Both are frequently used in upbringing, education, and care and work situations.

Weinstein conducted three experiments to investigate the extent to which a coercive way of speaking evokes resistance and thus undermines freedom of choice and free will (Weinstein *et al.*, 2020). The experiments provided evidence that speakers who used coercive language were perceived to be exerting more pressure, as well as being less supportive, and evoked resistance reactions among listeners. They also showed that a coercive style was the most important predictor of resistance. Furthermore, the semantics (meaning of words) and prosody (tone of voice) used appeared to communicate coercion and elicit resistance. For example, it may be coercive to repeatedly and emphatically try to convince the patient of the usefulness of an exercise. Conclusion: a coercive content and tone in the physiotherapist's style elicit resistance.

The coach's guiding conversation style has been developed in 'motivational interviewing', which has been applied increasingly in healthcare over the last 15 years. More research is also becoming available which substantiates the importance of motivational interviewing (Lundahl *et al.*, 2013; Morton *et al.*, 2015). For example, motivational interviewing have been proven highly effective in, among other things, quitting smoking (Harris *et al.*, 2010), maintaining body weight (Groeneveld *et al.*, 2010), taking more exercise (Lohmann *et al.*, 2010), and in patients with (chronic) pain (Alperstein & Sharpe, 2016).

More evidence on motivational interviewing can be found in the book by Miller and Rollnick (2012), in which a full chapter is devoted to the scientific foundation of this.

Often the question is whether motivational interviewing can also be applied to people with impaired cognitive abilities or people with cognitive dysfunctions (such as acquired brain injury). Of course, adaptation in the application of motivational strategies and techniques is necessary (Suarez, 2011), such as giving more structure to the conversation by summarising more often; supporting the patient more strongly in expressing their thoughts, feelings, and motives through reflections and using open questions that already give more direction; or using semi-closed questions. With these modifications, it is possible to effectively use motivational interviewing with patients with an acquired brain injury (Sherer *et al.*, 2007).

TARGETS FOR CHANGE

The targets for change that people have chosen themselves and in which they are guided by a physiotherapist are more often actually achieved (and are more relevant) than targets that the therapist has devised and given to the patient. This principle is based on the Goal Setting Theory of Latham and Locke (2007). Miller and Rollnick (2012) and Bandura (1994) have made it clear that self-regulation plays an important role in this, and that targets, reasons, motives, and necessity should primarily be elicited by the patient themselves instead of being told or imposed.

ADHERENCE

In science, a lot of research is done on 'adherence', as for example in the systematic review of McLean *et al.* (2010). A synonym for adherence is 'compliance'. The latter concept, in view of developments such as shared decision-making and motivational interviewing in which the patient's choice is central, not that of the care worker, is no longer entirely appropriate in this day and age. Nevertheless, the research remains relevant and interesting. McLean's review makes it clear that patients very often do not do what the coach advises them to do, but also often do not do what they themselves say they want to do.

McLean's recommendations to physiotherapists are therefore: (1) pay great attention to obstacles in the implementation of the patient's intentions; (2) be creative in responding to the patient's wishes; and (3) have access to a wide variety of therapy strategies, such as in the role of coach, to help the patient strengthen their motivation and sustainably change their behaviour.

A Cochrane review of adherence in chronic musculoskeletal pain studied a total of 42 trials, mainly in patients with spine-related pain and knee pain (Jordan *et al.*, 2010). The advice of the authors: tailor the exercises to the patient, scrupulously taking into account the patient's personal preferences; use simple behavioural and educational strategies, such as giving feedback and using a contract/arrangement; practice regularly under supervision; follow up with the confirmation of adequate practice; and support with resources (audio, video, photo, written instruction) to ensure this.

KNOWLEDGE AND BEHAVIOURAL CHANGE

The fact that knowledge influences behaviour and also promotes behavioural change in patients is widely accepted. Yet knowledge is often not enough. A study by Sherman on the follow-up of risk management advice by patients with lymphoedema after breast cancer showed that, despite sufficient knowledge, patients often did not follow the advice given to them. For example, highlighting the negative consequences of lymphoedema did not contribute to the patients' following of the advice. Instead, a guiding style, focused on the benefits of preventive measures, proved to have a positive effect (Sherman & Koelmeyer, 2013).

CHAPTER 22

The Role of Communicative Detective

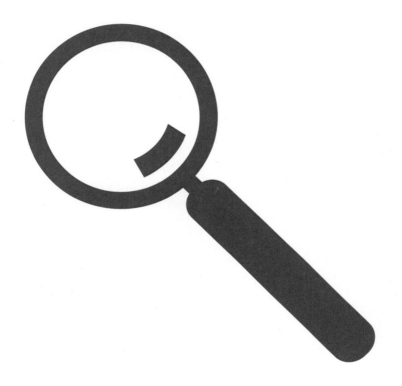

The communicative detective is the investigating and analysing professional who simultaneously collaborates and communicates with the patient. Research into shared decision-making ties in with this role, just like research into illness perceptions, the patient's use of words, the importance of psychosocial aspects in communication, and the view of the physiotherapist. This chapter gives a selection of the research into these subjects.

SHARED DECISION-MAKING

Glyn Elwyn is a well-known author in the field of shared decision-making (SDM). Together with Adrian Edwards, he has written several publications and also a book about SDM (Edwards & Elwyn, 2009). Although the book does not specifically deal with the paramedical or physiotherapy context, it certainly contains relevant chapters. Indeed, Elwyn's 'talk model' is the basis for working as a communicative detective.

There is a lot of discussion in the literature about SDM. Shay examined the patient's perceptions regarding this question (Shay & Lafata, 2014). Conclusion: even simple interactions are labelled as 'shared' by patients as long as there is agreement, attunement, and equivalence. This turns out to be more important than following the exact steps described for SDM in the literature. Of course, these steps are certainly helpful for the novice professional, but in the end, cooperation and agreement are the most important aspects to bear in mind.

That SDM is not only about decision-making with regard to the treatment, but also about diagnostic choices, is evident from the opinion-forming article by Polaris and Katz (2014). Their vision has been extrapolated in this book in the sharing of information with the patient regarding interim conclusions about the clinical reasoning process, while taking the medical history, and during the physical examination.

Incidentally, the arguments for applying SDM do not necessarily stem from the fact that SDM leads to a better outcome for therapy (Beasley et al., 2016). In the medical world, research on the outcome of SDM gives a mixed picture, but in the area of physiotherapy, relevant research is unfortunately very limited. For this reason, research in the medical setting (including general practitioner care) is used here. In the guiding principles of this book, autonomy has been formulated as a central value of the physiotherapy support to be provided. SDM clearly seems to make a positive contribution in this respect (Edwards & Elwyn, 2009; Stiggelbout et al., 2015; Oshima et al., 2013). This outweighs the importance of the lack of a positive outcome.

SDM is also easy to apply in the context of children and young people—with or without their parents (Butz et al., 2007). According to Butz's literature study, the involvement of a child can be increased through the use of various techniques: visual support (such as pictures, colouring books, dolls, dollhouses, etc.), taking turns (parents take a turn, followed by the child), teaching the child how to ask about things when they do not understand something, inviting the child to recount what they have understood, or role play to teach the child communication skills (in which the child, for example, takes the role of the physiotherapist and vice versa, or teaching the child to ask the physiotherapist a question in the role play). Feenstra and colleagues concluded on the basis of a systematic review that, in general, children from eight years of age can participate to a greater or lesser extent in decision-making (Feenstra et al., 2014). In most cases, this improves accordance between parents and child, as well as the quality of the overall decision-making process. At the same time, satisfaction with the decision often increases. SDM is also appropriate in the context of older people and informal carers (Pel-Littel & van Veenendaal, 2015).

With regard to the application of SDM in healthcare, there is also a bottleneck: care workers indicate that they want to apply SDM and embrace what it aims to achieve, but they often end up being unable to achieve SDM in the consultation room (Stiggelbout et al., 2015). This is also the case in physiotherapy, according to a study by Dierckx and colleagues (2013). Many physiotherapists believe that they apply SDM, but measurements of the patient's actual participation in the consultation do not show this at all: in many cases, participation is low to very low.

The use of PROs (patient-reported outcomes)—tools which measure the improvements in health experienced by the patient—seems to be helpful because it involves patients more in drawing up the treatment plan and monitoring its results. It also supports the care worker in their communication with the patient about this (Yang et al., 2018).

For people with limited health literacy skills, making decisions together with the physiotherapist is often more difficult. They are frequently inclined to ask fewer questions and participate less actively in the decision-making process. By taking this into account (e.g. by slowing down the pace, building a good relationship, stimulating the patient to ask questions, or using the teach-back method) the therapist can support the patient to fully participate in the decision-making process (Menendez et al., 2017).

SETTING TREATMENT GOALS

Scobbie has published on the setting of targets or goals, an activity of the communicative detective (Scobbie et al., 2013). Goal-setting is necessary in relation to the patient's self-management and is required to achieve patient-driven goals and assistance (Melin et al., 2019). It leads to greater patient involvement and commitment, because the goals are better understood and more relevant to the patient (Stevens et al., 2013). Stevens also links working with targets to the use of PROs, as mentioned in the Section "Shared decision-making". This can increase patient participation.

In a study with patients from a neurological rehabilitation unit, Holliday et al. (2007) investigated the usefulness of patient participation in setting treatment goals. Although the functional outcomes (improvement in activities) were not better or worse, it was clear that the patients experienced the goals as more relevant; moreover, they could express their autonomy more strongly and were more satisfied with the goals and goal-setting.

Research also shows that therapists often underestimate the number of skills they need to be able to perform goal-setting (Gardner et al., 2018). In addition, the same research revealed that therapists who have a more biomedical orientation seem to set their goals less in conjunction with the patient and also have consultations in which the patient becomes less involved.

COOPERATION IN EXAMINATION AND TREATMENT

A collaborative approach has become increasingly preferred within physiotherapy over the last 10 years. A case study that works out what this collaboration looks like in history taking, physical assessment, decision-making, and treatment is that of Edwin de Raaij (de Raaij et al., 2014). In his study, de Raaij clearly describes the importance of the patient's illness perceptions in relation to, among other things, decision-making and the formulation of treatment goals. Peter O'Sullivan's research group also published fascinating case studies in which this theme came to the fore (Bunzli et al., 2017; Caneiro et al., 2017).

O'Hagan did a qualitative study of the stories of patients with chronic pain. Once again, it turned out that the patients' illness perceptions strongly determine the behaviour they exhibit and that it can be difficult to determine the patient's perceptions. It is precisely for this reason that O'Hagan proposes an approach in which there is intensive cooperation with the patient (O'Hagan et al., 2013).

In order to discover what really concerns the patient about their health, what worries and emotions they have, and what thoughts and perceptions are involved, simply asking questions is not enough. Reflective listening is necessary (Lang et al., 2000; O'Keeffe et al., 2016; Slade et al., 2009; Van Dyk et al., 2019). Numerous researchers argue that using open questions, reflecting, and summarising are crucial skills. The roles of confidant and communicative detective are interwoven here.

ILLNESS PERCEPTIONS

An important model in this book is Leventhal's Common Sense Model of Illness Behaviour. This model describes how the patient forms cognitive and emotional beliefs about a health problem. The cognitive perceptions, often called illness perceptions, appear to have a strong relationship with the behaviour of the person concerned (Cameron & Leventhal, 2003). As the communicative detective goes through the diagnostic process with the patient, illness perceptions are always central, regardless of whether they are explicit or implicit. Leventhal's model has been subjected to a great deal of research, which Hagger, among others, has summarised in a meta-analysis (Hagger & Orbell, 2003). Hagger investigated 45 empirical studies in which more than 6,000 people were studied. The conclusions included that the model establishes a logical relationship between illness perceptions and behaviour. He also concluded that in patients with diabetes, heart failure, HIV, COPD, arthritis, breast cancer, and multiple sclerosis, the perception of a long (chronic) timeline and/or serious consequences correlates with avoidance behaviour. Foster and colleagues demonstrated this in a study of more than 1,500 patients with lower back pain (Foster *et al.*, 2008). The study also showed that the patient's perception of back pain as being more difficult to control and/or influence leads to a poorer prognosis.

Van Wilgen interviewed 27 patients with musculoskeletal pain (van Wilgen *et al.*, 2014). The interviews clearly showed how patients' illness perceptions determine their behaviour. It is therefore essential for the therapist to know the patient's illness perceptions so that they can take them into account and discuss them with the patient in order to influence their illness perceptions in a favourable direction. Van Wilgen's conclusion was therefore that the integration of illness perceptions into daily therapy practice is essential.

Illness perceptions are strongly linked to language and vocabulary, both on the part of the therapist and on the part of the patient. In Chapter 20, the physiotherapist's use of words was already discussed on the basis of the concept of 'nocebo'.

In line with this, the question immediately arises: How do you explain the diagnosis clearly to the patient? First of all, try to connect adequately with the patient by listening carefully to them (and making this obvious), acknowledging their feelings and thoughts, and allowing your explanations to fit in with their life experience and perceptions (Kilkku *et al.*, 2003). Provide information simply, clearly, and point by point; use simple language and words (Shaw *et al.*, 2009). Support the patient with written information in addition to the verbal information you provide (Gaston & Mitchell, 2005). Ask the patient if they would like additional information from you and what that might be (Reynolds *et al.*, 1981).

THE PATIENT'S USE OF WORDS

The words used by patients reveal a lot about their illness perceptions. It is important for the physiotherapist to realise that patients often form unrealistic and prognostically unfavourable perceptions of, for example, lower back pain (Darlow *et al.*, 2015). Darlow's qualitative research shows clearly that patient perceptions can only be measured to a limited extent with questionnaires, and that the real essence of the matter often only comes to the fore by listening carefully and reflecting with the patient on their perceptions and the consequences they attach to them in relation to their behaviour.

Patients' statements about their feelings, their obstacles, and their pain are often laced with metaphors. Lakoff argued that if patients want to say something about the obstacles they experience—their feelings and thoughts about their health and the pain they feel and what they think about it—they almost always and almost completely express themselves in metaphors (Lakoff & Johnson, 1980). Using simple words to actually describe these things is inadequate. What remains is the sketching of an image, a metaphor. 'If I bend my knee, it locks' is such statement. The patient experiences that their knee cannot move any further and describes this as 'locking'; this is what it feels like for them: something is holding them back. Or they might say, 'I feel a stabbing pain occasionally, deep inside'. The patient experiences a (painful) sensation that reminds them of and evokes the image of 'stabbing'. The patient uses words that describe what it looks like to them, and uses metaphors for this purpose. Physiotherapists do this too. The trick is to 'uncover' the patient's metaphor: to help the patient understand what they mean and what associations they make with it in terms of recovery. Furthermore, the physiotherapist themselves will want to use those metaphors, for example in providing education and advice, evoking an image that supports the patient's recovery.

An interesting book that provides a further insight into the world of the patient in pain is that by David Biro, a care worker and himself suffering from chronic pain (Malani, 2010). In this context, Joletta Belton's blog is also very interesting. Belton writes about her chronic pain, as well as her experiences in healthcare (Belton, 2020). A more scientific publication that also provides insight into the world of the patient in pain is Lennard Voogt's highly readable PhD research (2009), *The Emotional and Cognitive World of Patients with Chronic Pain*. His thesis includes qualitative research with people with chronic pain.

PSYCHOSOCIAL ASPECTS

The question arises whether physiotherapists adequately include psychosocial aspects in their consultations, such as by thoroughly 'examining' patients' illness perceptions and topics like stress, behaviour, and lifestyle. Research by Oostendorp (Oostendorp & Duquet, 2010) showed that many physiotherapists take a biomedical history as well as conducting a biomedically oriented examination, then continue with their treatment in this way. A study by van Wilgen yielded similar results (van Wilgen *et al.*, 2014). It also turns out that physiotherapists often find it difficult to address psychosocial aspects in the conversation with the patient. They often leave it to come up by chance or omit it completely (Bastiaenen, 2010).

Stress plays a role in many health problems: sometimes causal, sometimes as an inhibitor to recovery, sometimes both. Physiotherapists probably often miss this possibility with their patients. However, this phenomenon is well known to general practitioners (Noordman *et al.*, 2007). Noordman's publication showed that two-thirds of patients who thought their complaints were related to stress did not discuss this during the consultation with the GP. So patients often don't bring it up themselves and the care worker often fails to do so. This likely also applies to physiotherapists. As an extension of this study, a review by Derksen and Bensing is interesting (Derksen *et al.*, 2013). This review of the power of empathy shows that there is a positive correlation between empathy and (1) patient satisfaction, (2) patient involvement in the consultation, and (3) anxiety and distress levels. In other words, the attitude of an empathic clinician makes it possible for the patient to bring up difficult themes such as stress more easily and more often.

Verheul (2008) showed that a care worker with a warm, empathic attitude, combined with the establishment of positive expectations regarding recovery, is important. In patients with severe menstrual pain, the doctor's attitude was found to positively correlate with a reduction in the patient's anxiety. A study by Acquati *et al.* (2019) showed that the more empathic the osteopath is, the better the results in terms of the degree of pain the patient experiences in the course of the treatment. This is a relevant observation for physiotherapists, who regularly see patients who also have anxious and catastrophic thoughts about their state of health and/or pain.

THE PHYSIOTHERAPIST'S VIEWS

The therapist's views or perceptions are also important. Many therapists have a biomedical view on musculoskeletal pain, whereas much of the literature argues that a biopsychosocial view on musculoskeletal pain is helpful (Houben *et al.*, 2005; Hasenbring *et al.*, 2012; Waddell, 2004). A biomedical view can harm the recovery of a patient with persistent pain (Domenech *et al.*, 2011). Internationally, the biopsychosocial view on health problems is seen as fundamental (Engel, 1977; Adler, 2009).

The actual view of the physiotherapist can be examined with the aid of tools specifically designed for this purpose, such as the Pain Attitudes and Beliefs Scale for Physiotherapists (with regard to attitude and views on chronic pain management) and the Health Care Providers' Pain and Impairment Relationship Scale, which provides a good picture of the therapist's attitudes and views with regard to functional expectations in patients with chronic lower back pain.

EFFICIENCY

It is often argued that adding personal care, making space for the patient and their story, personal attention and emotional involvement, to the biomedical elements of a consultation or treatment is time-consuming and conflicts with productivity. One would simply rule out the other. Yet this is a myth. Boffeli and colleagues researched the connection between productivity and patient experiences (Boffeli *et al.*, 2012). Their conclusion was clear: there are many care workers who succeed both in being productive and in building a warm and personal relationship with patients, as well as paying ample attention to the aspects that are important to the patient and giving a good explanation of those elements that the patient wants.

We again refer to a final publication in the National Voice anthology, *Prioritising Person-Centred Care, Supporting Shared Decision-Making* (2014). This is a synthesis that includes a total of 48 scientific reviews and studies about the application and improvement of decision-making in the consultation room, such as strengthening patient participation in weighing up pros and cons, making decisions together, and so on.

CHAPTER 23

The Role of Teacher

The role of a teacher is aimed at 'making the patient wiser'. The teacher provides information and education. That is why in this chapter, among other things, we again look at evidence regarding cognitive psychology. Important here is the extent to which patients withhold information and the effect this has on their behaviour (thinking and acting). In addition to as the physiotherapist's beliefs, the relationship with the patient plays an important role in this.

Pain neuroscience education provision is commonly applied in physiotherapy. That is why a section is devoted to it in this chapter.

COGNITIVE PSYCHOLOGY AND EDUCATION PROVISION

It is a fact that our behaviour is influenced and partly determined by our thoughts. Cognitive psychology has demonstrated this more than once (Chomsky, 1957; Ellis, 1962). Making causal connections is a natural response for humans. The studies on the value of the Common Sense model (see also Chapter 22) make this clear (Hagger & Orbell, 2003). As a result, influencing patients' thoughts through information and education provision is an important strategy.

In advance of providing information and education, it is advisable to get the patient to pay attention to the matter of 'being open'. Is the patient ready for and interested in the information you want to give? In motivational interviewing, in order to facilitate this, the patient is asked for permission beforehand. Although the literature is not entirely clear on this matter, it seems to have added value (Fletcher et al., 2019; Sullivan et al., 2019; Wijma et al., 2016).

When providing information or education, the following focal points emerge from the literature (Kilkku et al., 2003; Louw & Puentedura, 2013; Mosley & Butler, 2017; Ogden, 2019; Shaw et al., 2009; Talevski et al., 2020):

- Use a good structure; a lot of information requires more structure and well-considered steps;
- Tell the patient the most important things first (primacy effect);
- Simplify your information; do not use jargon unless absolutely necessary;
- Be concrete;
- Don't tell the patient too much (you may even err on the side of 'too little');
- Connect to the patient's world so that the information is meaningful;
- Repeat, using slightly different words;
- Support your explanations with written information;
- Use the 'teach back' technique at the end;
- Return to your previous explanation in the next consultation.

Of course, the use of photographs, drawings, diagrams, and pictograms can support the provision of information and education. Selectively and purposefully used, such aids help the patient to understand and remember. The amount of detail should preferably be limited (Houts et al., 2006). If possible, try to let the patient feel or experience (parts of) your explanation (Mosley & Butler, 2017; Peper et al., 2013; Vibe Fersum et al., 2013). Of course, you should also be vigilant about the words you use—the nocebo effect is lurking (Chapter 20).

REMEMBERING INFORMATION

An important question is: What is the connection between therapy compliance and what the patient remembers from the therapist's explanation? Linn did research on this in patients with intestinal inflammation (Linn et al., 2013). She found that remembering explanations correlated positively with medication intake in the patients studied. Incidentally, it turned out that on average, the patients only remembered half of the explanations they were given. Remembering information can be improved by using the teach-back method (Roberts et al., 2016; Talevski et al., 2020).

PAIN NEUROSCIENCE EDUCATION PROVISION

Much research has been done on the effect of education provision in patients with chronic musculoskeletal pain. A systematic review by Louw and colleagues concluded that there is strong evidence that education provision about the neurophysiology and neurobiology of pain has a positive effect on pain, limitations in activities, catastrophising, and physical functioning (Louw et al., 2011). In the case of poorly understood complaints or medically inexplicable complaints, the importance of education provision has been emphasised by the literature research of Weiland et al. (2012). Responding to and understanding the patient's expectations enables the care worker to influence the patient's illness perceptions about education provision; it also reduces anxiety and improves patient satisfaction. Good explanations reduce symptoms. A patient-focused and positive or warm interaction style reduces the need for care and improves the patient's coping ability. If you are sincerely interested and attentive to the doubts and insecurities of the patient, they will accept the message far more readily (Sullivan et al., 2019).

In patients with pain, physiotherapists can successfully use a cognitive behavioural approach through education provision. In Archer's small study of fibromyalgia patients, improvements were found in the areas of fear of movement, pain catastrophising, depressive symptoms, pain, and disabilities; these improvements still existed at follow-up after six months (Archer et al., 2013).

THE RELATIONSHIP

In his book on education provision and teaching, Marzano makes a plea for the development of a good relationship between the teacher and the student. According to his research, the learning results are then clearly better (Marzano & Kendall, 2006). It seems logical that this also applies in physiotherapy.

THINKING AND DOING

Physiotherapists often combine giving patients education with letting them gain experience, mostly through doing exercises. This is an operant approach combined with a cognitive approach. Peper and colleagues developed an interesting argument based on two cases, focusing on the following core aspects: (1) the words you use are important, just like those already used when talking to the patient; (2) let the patient experience what you have explained to them (cognitively) wherever possible, which makes the message considerably more powerful—biofeedback can help here; and (3) dare to be creative and tackle things differently to others (Peper et al., 2013). Caneiro et al. and O'Sullivan et al. (Caneiro et al., 2017; O'Sullivan et al., 2018) also showed in studies with patients with lower back pain that a combination of operant, cognitive, and motivational techniques can positively influence lower back pain.

THE BELIEFS OF THE PHYSIOTHERAPIST

The beliefs of the physiotherapist when providing education seem to make a difference. Inadvertently and/or unintentionally, therapists often transfer their own illness perceptions to patients, such as by suggesting that one 'carefully' increase the load (Barsky, 2017). A study by Ferrari showed that (pain) self-efficacy and fear of movement are associated with pain intensity and disability in people with chronic lower back pain (Ferrari et al., 2015). The authors indicate that it may be the physiotherapists themselves who stimulate avoidance behaviour in patients through well-intentioned predictions of failure and avoidance advice. What we want to avoid or remove, we subconsciously reinforce. Lakke's dissertation (2014) also showed that the attitudes of physiotherapists have unintended effects. Physiotherapists with a stronger fear of movement negatively influenced their subjects, which led to the subjects showing a poorer performance on a capacity test.

And last but not least, another reference to the National Voices publication *Prioritising Person-Centred Care. Improving Information and Understanding* (2014). This is a synthesis, which includes a total of 85 scientific reviews and studies, on the improvement of patient information and education, such as tailored education, digital support for patient information, and more.

Acquati, A, Uberti, S, Aquino, A., Cerasetti, E., Castagna, C., Rovere-Querini, P., & Pisa, V. (2019). Do empathic osteopaths achieve better clinical results? An observational feasibility study. *International Journal of Osteopathic Medicine, 32*, 2–6.

Adler, R. H. (2009). Engel's biopsychosocial model is still relevant today. *Journal of Psychosomatic Research, 67* (6), 607–611.

Ahlsen, B., Mengshoel, A. M., Bondevik, H., & Engebretsen, E. (2018). Physiotherapists as detectives: Investigating clues and plots in the clinical encounter. *Medical Humanities, 44* (1), 40–45.

Alperstein, D., & Sharpe, L. (2016). The efficacy of motivational interviewing in adults with chronic pain: A meta-analysis and systematic review. *The Journal of Pain, 17* (4), 393–403.

American Psychiatric Association. (2013). *Diagnostic and statistical manual of mental disorders (DSM-5®)*. American Psychiatric Pub.

Archer, K. R., Motzny, N., Abraham, C. M., Yaffe, D., Seebach, C. L., Devin, C. J., Spengler, D. M., McGirt, M. J., Aaronson, O. S., & Cheng, J. S. (2013). Cognitive-behavioral–based physical therapy to improve surgical spine outcomes: A case series. *Physical Therapy, 93* (8), 1130–1139.

Australian Commission on Safety and Quality in Health Care. (2015). *Health literacy: Taking action to improve safety and quality*. Australian Commission on Safety and Quality in Health Care.

Baart, A. (2003). The fragile power of listening. *Practical Theology in South Africa (Praktiese Teologie in Suid-Afrika), 18* (3), 136–156.

Bandura, A. (1994). *Self-efficacy*. Wiley Online Library.

Bandura, A. (2010). Self-efficacy. *The Corsini encyclopedia of psychology*, 1–3.

Barsky, A. J. (2017). The iatrogenic potential of the physician's words. *JAMA, 318* (24), 2425–2426.

Bassett, S. F. (2003). The assessment of patient adherence to physiotherapy rehabilitation. *New Zealand Journal of Physiotherapy, 31* (2), 60–66.

Bastemeijer, C. M., Voogt, L., van Ewijk, J. P., & Hazelzet, J. A. (2016). What do patient values and preferences mean? A taxonomy based on a systematic review of qualitative papers. *Patient Education and Counseling, 100* (5), 871-881. doi: 10.1016/j.pec.2016.12.019.

Bastiaenen, C. H. G. (2010). Waarom volgen we onze richtlijnen…niet? *Nederlands tijdschrift voor Fysiotherapie, 4* (120), 144–155.

Beasley, M., Jones, E., McBeth, J., Jones, G. T., Hannaford, P., Lovell, K., Symmons, D., Keeley, P., Woby, S., & Prescott, G. (2016). 162 receiving preferred treatment not associated with positive outcome in a randomized trial. *Rheumatology, 55* (suppl_1), i127–i127.

Belton, J. (2020). My Cuppa Jo. Making sense of pain through science and stories. Bridging the gap between patients and health professionals. [Blog]. *My Cuppa Jo*. http://www.mycuppajo.com

Benedetti, F. (2002). How the doctor's words affect the patient's brain. *Evaluation & the Health Professions, 25* (4), 369–386.

Benedetti, F. (2013). Placebo and the new physiology of the doctor-patient relationship. *Physiological reviews, 93* (3), 1207–1246.

Benedetti, F., Carlino, E., & Piedimonte, A. (2016a). Increasing uncertainty in CNS clinical trials: The role of placebo, nocebo, and Hawthorne effects. *The Lancet Neurology, 15* (7), 736–747.

Benedetti, F., Frisaldi, E., Carlino, E., Giudetti, L., Pampallona, A., Zibetti, M., Lanotte, M., & Lopiano, L. (2016b). Teaching neurons to respond to placebos. *The Journal of Physiology, 594* (19), 5647–5660.

Benedetti, F., Thoen, W., Blanchard, C., Vighetti, S., & Arduino, C. (2013). Pain as a reward: Changing the meaning of pain from negative to positive co-activates opioid and cannabinoid systems. *Pain, 154* (3), 361–367.

Bijma, M. (2012). Gedragsverandering voor de fysiotherapeut—Deel 2: Therapietrouw. *Physios, Deel 2: therapietrouw*.

Boardman, H. F., Thomas, E., Millson, D. S., & Croft, P. (2005). Psychological, sleep, lifestyle, and comorbid associations with headache. *Headache: The Journal of Head and Face Pain, 45* (6), 657–669.

Bodai, B. I., Nakata, T. E., Wong, W. T., Clark, D. R., Lawenda, S., Tsou, C., Liu, R., Shiue, L., Cooper, N., & Rehbein, M. (2018). Lifestyle medicine: A brief review of its dramatic impact on health and survival. *The Permanente Journal, 22,* 17–025.

Boffeli, T. J., Thongvanh, K. L., Evans, S. J. H., & Ahrens, C. R. (2012). Patient experience and physician productivity: Debunking the mythical divide at HealthPartners clinics. *The Permanente Journal, 16* (4), 19.

Brinjikji, W., Luetmer, P., Comstock, B., Bresnahan, B. W., Chen, L., Deyo, R., Halabi, S., Turner, J. A., Avins, A., & James, K. (2015). Systematic literature review of imaging features of spinal degeneration in asymptomatic populations. *American Journal of Neuroradiology, 36* (4), 811–816.

Brown, B. (2013). *The Power of Vulnerability: Teachings on Authenticity, Connection, and Courage.* Louisville: Sounds True.

Brun-Cottan, N., McMillian, D., & Hastings, J. (2018). Defending the art of physical therapy: Expanding inquiry and crafting culture in support of therapeutic alliance. *Physiotherapy Theory and Practice, 36,* 1–10.

Brunner, E., Dankaerts, W., O'Sullivan, K., Meichtry, A., Bauer, C., & Probst, M. (2019). Associations between alliance, physiotherapists' confidence in managing the patient and patient-reported distress in chronic low back pain practice. *European Journal of Physiotherapy, 21,* 1–5.

Bunzli, S., Smith, A., Schütze, R., Lin, I., & O'Sullivan, P. (2017). Making sense of low back pain and pain-related fear. *Journal of Orthopaedic & Sports Physical Therapy, 47* (9), 628–636.

Burns, J. W., & Evon, D. (2007). Common and specific process factors in cardiac rehabilitation: Independent and interactive effects of the working alliance and self-efficacy. *Health Psychology, 26* (6), 684.

Butler, D. (2013). *Course syllabus "Explain Pain".* NOI.

Butler, D. S., & Moseley, G. L. (2013). *Explain Pain,* 2nd Edn. Noigroup Publications.

Butz, A. M., Walker, J. M., Pulsifer, M., & Winkelstein, M. (2007). Shared decision making in school-age children with asthma. *Pediatric Nursing, 33* (2), 111.

Cameron, L. D., & Leventhal, H. (2003). *The self-regulation of health and illness behaviour.* Psychology Press.

Caneiro, J., Smith, A., Rabey, M., Moseley, G. L., & O'Sullivan, P. (2017). Process of change in pain-related fear: Clinical insights from a single case report of persistent back pain managed with cognitive functional therapy. *Journal of Orthopaedic & Sports Physical Therapy, 47* (9), 637–651.

Carkhuff, R. R. (1969). *Helping and human relations: A primer for lay and professional leaders,* vol. 1. New York: Holt, Reinhardt, and Winston.

CBO, Zorgmodule Zelfmanagement 1.0. (2014). CBO.

Chomsky, N. (1957). *Syntactic structures.* New York: de Gruyter.

Chugh, U., Agger-Gupta, N., Dillmann, E., Fisher, D., Gronnerud, P., Kulig, J., Kurtz, S., & Stenhouse, A. (1994). The case of culturally sensitive health care: A comparative study of health beliefs related to culture in six north-east Calgary communities. *Calgary, AB: Citizenship & Heritage Secretariat, Alberta Community Development, & Calgary Catholic Immigration Society.*

Cohen, S., Janicki-Deverts, D., & Miller, G. E. (2007). Psychological stress and disease. *JAMA, 298* (14), 1685–1687.

Cole, S. A., & Bird, J. (2013). *The medical interview e-book: The three-function approach.* Elsevier Health Sciences.

Commonwealth of Australia. (2009a). *Communicating with people who are blind or have vision impairment factsheet.* Australian Government. Department of Families, Housing, Community Services and Indigenous Affairs. http://resources.fahcsia.gov.au/ConsumerTrainingSupportProducts/employers/blind_vision.htm

Commonwealth of Australia. (2009b). *Communicating with people who are deaf or have hearing impairment factsheet.* Australian Government. Department of Families, Housing, Community Services and Indigenous Affairs. http://hearingservices.gov.au/wps/poc/hso?1dmy&urile=wcm%3apath%3a/HSO+Content/Public/Home/For+Everyone/FactsheetsAndForms/

Communicatietips. (2015a). [Voorlichting en educatie]. *Hoorwijzer.nl NVVS.* https://www.hoorwijzer.nl/hoorhulpmiddelen/overige-hulpmiddelen/communicatietips.html

Communicatietips. (2015b). [Voorlichting / educatie]. *Leren.nl / Stichting Plotsdoven.* http://www.leren.nl/cursus/sociale-vaardigheden/bijzondere-mensen/slechthorenden-en-doven.html

Compernolle, T. (1999). *Stress, friend and foe: Vital stress management at work and home.* Synergo, The Hague.

Cooper, C., & Quick, J. C. (2017). *The handbook of stress and health: A guide to research and practice.* New York: John Wiley & Sons.

Cooper, K., Smith, B. H., & Hancock, E. (2009). Patients' perceptions of self-management of chronic low back pain: Evidence for enhancing patient education and support. *Physiotherapy, 95* (1), 43–50.

Cuyul-Vásquez, I., Barría, J. A., Perez, N. F., & Fuentes, J. (2019). The influence of verbal suggestions in the management of musculoskeletal pain: A narrative review. *Physical Therapy Reviews, 24* (3–4), 175–181.

Darlow, B., Dean, S., Perry, M., Mathieson, F., Baxter, G. D., & Dowell, A. (2015). Easy to harm, hard to heal: Patient views about the back. *Spine, 40* (11), 842–850.

Darlow, B., Dowell, A., Baxter, G. D., Mathieson, F., Perry, M., & Dean, S. (2013). The enduring impact of what clinicians say to people with low back pain. *The Annals of Family Medicine, 11* (6), 527–534.

de Raaij, E. J., Pool, J., Maissan, F., & Wittink, H. (2014). Illness perceptions and activity limitations in osteoarthritis of the knee: A case report intervention study. *Manual Therapy, 19* (2), 169–172.

de Ridder, D., & Schreurs, K. (2001). Developing interventions for chronically ill patients: Is coping a helpful concept? *Clinical Psychology Review, 21* (2), 205–240.

Deber, R. B., Kraetschmer, N., Urowitz, S., & Sharpe, N. (2005). Patient, consumer, client, or customer: What do people want to be called? *Health Expectations, 8* (4), 345–351.

Deci, E. L., & Vansteenkiste, M. (2004). Self-determination theory and basic need satisfaction: Understanding human development in positive psychology. *Ricerche di Psicologia, 27* (1), 23–40.

Demarais, A., & White, V. (2007). *First impressions: What you don't know about how others see you.* New York: Bantam.

Derksen, F., Bensing, J., & Lagro-Janssen, A. (2013). Effectiveness of empathy in general practice: A systematic review. *British Journal of General Practice, 63* (606), e76–e84.

Di Blasi, Z., Harkness, E., Ernst, E., Georgiou, A., & Kleijnen, J. (2001). Influence of context effects on health outcomes: A systematic review. *The Lancet, 357* (9258), 757–762.

Dierckx, K., Deveugele, M., Roosen, P., & Devisch, I. (2013). Implementation of shared decision making in physical therapy: Observed level of involvement and patient preference. *Physical Therapy, 93* (10), 1321–1330.

Dijksterhuis, A. (2011). *Het slimme onbewuste.* Amsterdam: Prometheus.

Dilts, R. B., & Grinder, J. (1980). *Neuro-Linguistic Programming.* Meta. https://books.google.nl/books?id=7kCdswEACAAJ

Doll, R., Peto, R., Boreham, J., & Sutherland, I. (2004). Mortality in relation to smoking: 50 years' observations on male British doctors. *BMJ, 328* (7455), 1519.

Domenech, J., Sánchez-Zuriaga, D., Segura-Ortí, E., Espejo-Tort, B., & Lisón, J. (2011). Impact of biomedical and biopsychosocial training sessions on the attitudes, beliefs, and recommendations of health care providers about low back pain: A randomised clinical trial. *Pain, 152* (11), 2557–2563.

Donaghy, M. E., & Morss, K. (2000). Guided reflection: A framework to facilitate and assess reflective practice within the discipline of physiotherapy. *Physiotherapy Theory and Practice, 16* (1), 3–14.

Duncan, B. L., & Miller, S. D. (2000). *The heroic client: Doing client-directed, outcome-informed therapy.* New York: Jossey-Bass.

Edwards, A., & Elwyn, G. (2009). *Shared decision-making in health care: Achieving evidence-based patient choice.* Oxford: Oxford University Press.

Ellis, A. (1962). *Reason and emotion in psychotherapy,* 1st ed. New York: Lyle Stuart.

Elwyn, G., Tsulukidze, M., Edwards, A., Légaré, F., & Newcombe, R. (2013). Using a 'talk' model of shared decision making to propose an observation-based measure: Observer OPTION 5 Item. *Patient Education and Counseling, 93* (2), 265–271.

Engel, G. L. (1977). The need for a new medical model: A challenge for biomedicine. *Science, 196* (4286), 129–136.

Engers, A. J., Jellema, P., Wensing, M., van der Windt, D. A., Grol, R., & van Tulder, M. W. (2008). Individual patient education for low back pain. *Cochrane Database of Systematic Review, 1* (CD004057). doi: 10.1002/14651858.CD004057.pub3.

Epstein, R. M., Alper, B. S., & Quill, T. E. (2004). Communicating evidence for participatory decision making. *Jama, 291* (19), 2359–2366.

Essential competency profile for physiotherapists in Canada. (2009). National Physiotherapy Advisory Group. https://physiotherapy.ca/sites/default/files/competency_profile_final_en_0.pdf

Evers, A. W., Colloca, L., Blease, C., Annoni, M., Atlas, L. Y., Benedetti, F., Bingel, U., Büchel, C., Carvalho, C., & Colagiuri, B. (2018). Implications of placebo and nocebo effects for clinical practice: Expert consensus. *Psychotherapy and Psychosomatics, 87* (4), 204–210.

Evers, A. W., Verhoeven, E. W., van Middendorp, H., Sweep, F. C., Kraaimaat, F. W., Donders, A. R. T., Eijsbouts, A. E., van Laarhoven, A. I., de Brouwer, S. J., & Wirken, L. (2014). Does stress affect the joints? Daily stressors, stress vulnerability, immune and HPA axis activity, and short-term disease and symptom fluctuations in rheumatoid arthritis. *Annals of the Rheumatic Diseases, 73* (9), 1683–1688.

Feenstra, B., Boland, L., Lawson, M. L., Harrison, D., Kryworuchko, J., Leblanc, M., & Stacey, D. (2014). Interventions to support children's engagement in health-related decisions: A systematic review. *BMC Pediatrics, 14* (1), 1.

Ferrari, S., Chiarotto, A., Pellizzer, M., Vanti, C., & Monticone, M. (2015). Pain self-efficacy and fear of movement are similarly associated with pain intensity and disability in Italian patients with chronic low back pain. *Pain Practice, 6* (8), 1040–1047. doi: 10.1111/papr.12397

Ferreira, P. H., Ferreira, M. L., Maher, C. G., Refshauge, K. M., Latimer, J., & Adams, R. D. (2013). The therapeutic alliance between clinicians and patients predicts outcome in chronic low back pain. *Physical Therapy, 93* (4), 470–478.

Fischhoff, B. (2012). *Communicating risks and benefits: An evidence-based user's guide.* Washington, DC: Government Printing Office.

Flaxman, S. R., Bourne, R. R., Resnikoff, S., Ackland, P., Braithwaite, T., Cicinelli, M. V., Das, A., Jonas, J. B., Keeffe, J., & Kempen, J. H. (2017). Global causes of blindness and distance vision impairment 1990–2020: A systematic review and meta-analysis. *The Lancet Global Health, 5* (12), e1221–e1234.

Fletcher, R., Braithwaite, F. A., Woodhouse, M., MacInnes, A., & Stanton, T. R. (2019). Does readiness to change influence pain-related outcomes after an educational intervention for people with chronic pain? A pragmatic, preliminary study. *Physiotherapy Theory and Practice, 35,* 1–12.

Folkman, S. (2011). *The Oxford handbook of stress, health, and coping.* Oxford: Oxford University Press.

Foster, N. E., Bishop, A., Thomas, E., Main, C., Horne, R., Weinman, J., & Hay, E. (2008). Illness perceptions of low back pain patients in primary care: What are they, do they change and are they associated with outcome? *Pain, 136* (1), 177–187.

Frankel, R. M., & Stein, T. (1999). Getting the most out of the clinical encounter: The four habits model. *The Permanente Journal, 3* (3), 79–88.

Gardner, T., Refshauge, K., McAuley, J., Hübscher, M., Goodall, S., & Smith, L. (2018). Goal setting practice in chronic low back pain. What is current practice and is it affected by beliefs and attitudes? *Physiotherapy Theory and Practice, 34* (10), 795–805.

Gaston, C. M., & Mitchell, G. (2005). Information giving and decision-making in patients with advanced cancer: A systematic review. *Social Science & Medicine, 61* (10), 2252–2264.

Gemeente Amsterdam. Onderzoek, Informatie en Statistiek. (2014). [Informatief]. *Gemeente Amsterdam.* http://www.ois.amsterdam.nl/nieuwsarchief/2014/amsterdam-groeit-door

Gillissen, F. (2014). Omgaan met Alzheimer. VUmc Alzheimercentrum [Educaties]. *NTR academie.* http://ntracademie.nl/cursussen/cursuspagina/10-stappencursus-omgaan-met-alzheimer/stap/intro.html

Gordon, T. (1977). *Leadership, Executive ability, Organizational behavior.* New York: Wyden Books. https://archive.org/details/leadereffectiven00gord/page/57

Groeneveld, I. F., Proper, K. I., van der Beek, A. J., & van Mechelen, W. (2010). Sustained body weight reduction by an individual-based lifestyle intervention for workers in the construction industry at risk for cardiovascular disease: Results of a randomized controlled trial. *Preventive Medicine, 51* (3), 240–246.

Grotle, M., Brox, J. I., Veierød, M. B., Glomsrød, B., Lønn, J. H., & Vøllestad, N. K. (2005). Clinical course and prognostic factors in acute low back pain: Patients consulting primary care for the first time. *Spine, 30* (8), 976–982.

Hagenaars, L. H., & Bos, J. (2010). *Over de kunst van hulpverlenen: Het meerdimensionale belasting-belastbaarheidsmodel: Een vakfilosofisch model voor een menswaardige gezondheidszorg.* NPI.

Hagger, M. S., & Orbell, S. (2003). A meta-analytic review of the common-sense model of illness representations. *Psychology and Health, 18* (2), 141–184.

Hall, A. M., Ferreira, P. H., Maher, C. G., Latimer, J., & Ferreira, M. L. (2010). The influence of the therapist-patient relationship on treatment outcome in physical rehabilitation: A systematic review. *Physical Therapy, 90* (8), 1099–1110. doi: 10.2522/ptj.20090245

Hall, J. A., Roter, D. L., & Katz, N. R. (1988). Meta-analysis of correlates of provider behavior in medical encounters. *Medical Care, 27* (7), 657–675.

Hall, J. A., Roter, D. L., & Rand, C. S. (1981). Communication of affect between patient and physician. *Journal of Health and Social Behavior, 22* (1), 18–30.

Harrigan, J. A., Oxman, T. E., & Rosenthal, R. (1985). Rapport expressed through nonverbal behavior. *Journal of Nonverbal Behavior, 9* (2), 95–110.

Harris, K. J., Catley, D., Good, G. E., Cronk, N. J., Harrar, S., & Williams, K. B. (2010). Motivational interviewing for smoking cessation in college students: A group randomized controlled trial. *Preventive Medicine, 51* (5), 387–393.

Hasenbring, M. I., Rusu, A. C., & Turk, D. C. (2012). *From acute to chronic back pain: Risk factors, mechanisms, and clinical implications.* Oxford: Oxford University Press.

Heerkens, Y., Hendriks, H., & De Graaf-Peters, V. (2012). KNGF-guideline record keeping in physical therapy. 2011. https://www. fysionetevidencebased. nl/index. php/richtlijnen/richtlijnen/ fysiotherapeutischeverslaglegging-2011.

Heneweer, H. (2011). *Correlates of low back pain: A closer look at physical activity, physical fitness and personal attributes.* https://limo.libis.be/primo-explore/search?sortby=rank&vid=Lirias&lang=nl_BE

Heritage, J., Robinson, J. D., Elliott, M. N., Beckett, M., & Wilkes, M. (2007). Reducing patients' unmet concerns in primary care: The difference one word can make. *Journal of General Internal Medicine, 22* (10), 1429–1433.

Herman, R. E., & Williams, K. N. (2009). Elderspeak's influence on resistiveness to care: Focus on behavioral events. *American Journal of Alzheimer's disease and Other Dementias, 24* (5), 417–423.

Hessel, J. A. (2009). Presence in nursing practice: A concept analysis. *Holistic Nursing Practice, 23* (5), 276–281.

Heyland, D. K., Allan, D. E., Rocker, G., Dodek, P., Pichora, D., & Gafni, A. (2009). Discussing prognosis with patients and their families near the end of life: Impact on satisfaction with end-of-life care. *Open Medicine, 3* (2), 101–110.

Hill, C. E., & Knox, S. (2001). Self-disclosure. *Psychotherapy: Theory, Research, Practice, Training, 38* (4), 413.

Hinz, C. A. (2000). *Communicating with your patients: Skills for building rapport.* American Medical Association.

Hirsch, A., Haskal, Z., Hertzer, N., Bakal, C., Creager, M., & Halperin, J. (2006). Practice Guidelines for the management of patients with peripheral arterial disease (lower extremity, renal, mesenteric, and abdominal aortic): A collaborative report from the American Association for Vascular Surgery/Society for Vascular Surgery, Society for Cardiovascular Angiography and Interventions, Society for Vascular Medicine and Biology, Society of Interventional Radiology, and the ACC/AHA Task Force on Practice Guidelines (Writing Committee to Develop Guidelines for the Management of Patients With Peripheral Arterial Disease): Endorsed by the American Association of Cardiovascular and Pulmonary Rehabilitation; National Heart, Lung, and Blood Institute; Society for Vascular Nursing; TransAtlantic Inter-Society Consensus; and Vascular Disease Foundation. *Circulation, 113* (11), 463–654.

Hofman, E. (2013). *Interculturele gespreksvoering: Theorie en praktijk van het TOPOI-model* (derde druk). Bohn Stafleu van Loghum.

Hollander, J., Derks, L., & Meijer, A. (1990). NLP in Nederland. *Utrecht/Antwerpen: Servire.*

Holliday, R. C., Cano, S., Freeman, J. A., & Playford, E. D. (2007). Should patients participate in clinical decision making? An optimised balance block design controlled study of goal setting in a rehabilitation unit. *Journal of Neurology, Neurosurgery & Psychiatry, 78* (6), 576–580.

Holmes, T. H., & Rahe, R. H. (1967). The social readjustment rating scale. *Journal of Psychosomatic Research, 11* (2), 213–218.

Horst, M., Lindeboom, R., & Lucas, C. (2005). De aanwezigheid van psychische problematiek in de eerstelijns fysiotherapiepraktijk: Een clusteranalyse. De prognostische waarde van de Vierdimensionale Klachtenlijst (4DKL). *Nederlands Tijdschrift voor Fysiotherapie, 115* (4), 106–111.

Houben, R., Gijsen, A., Peterson, J., De Jong, P., & Vlaeyen, J. (2005). Do health care providers' attitudes towards back pain predict their treatment recommendations? Differential predictive validity of implicit and explicit attitude measures. *Pain, 114* (3), 491–498.

Houts, P. S., Doak, C. C., Doak, L. G., & Loscalzo, M. J. (2006). The role of pictures in improving health communication: A review of research on attention, comprehension, recall, and adherence. *Patient Education and Counseling, 61* (2), 173–190.

Huber, M., Knottnerus, J. A., Green, L., van der Horst, H., Jadad, A. R., Kromhout, D., Leonard, B., Lorig, K., Loureiro, M. I., & van der Meer, J. W. (2011). How should we define health? *BMJ, 343,* d4163.

Jedeloo, S., & Weele, E. van. (2015). *Zorgbasics: Zelfmanagement* (2e druk). Boom Lemma.

Jordan, J. E., Buchbinder, R., & Osborne, R. H. (2010). Conceptualising health literacy from the patient perspective. *Patient Education and Counseling, 79* (1), 36–42.

Jordan, J. L., Holden, M. A., Mason, E., & Foster, N. E. (2010). Interventions to improve adherence to exercise for chronic musculoskeletal pain in adults. *Cochrane Database of Systematic Review, 1* (1), CD005956.

Keirse, M. (2011). *Helpen bij verlies en verdriet: Een gids voor het gezin en de hulpverlener*. Lannoo Meulenhoff-Belgium.

Kessler, R. C., Aguilar-Gaxiola, S., Alonso, J., Chatterji, S., Lee, S., & Üstün, T. B. (2009). The WHO world mental health (WMH) surveys. *Die Psychiatrie, 6* (01), 5–9.

Kilkku, N., Munnukka, T., & Lehtinen, K. (2003). From information to knowledge: The meaning of information-giving to patients who had experienced first-episode psychosis. *Journal of Psychiatric and Mental Health Nursing, 10* (1), 57–64.

King, J., Tessier, S., Charette, M.-J., & Gaudet, D. (2018). Patient education provided by physiotherapists for patients with chronic obstructive pulmonary disease: Results of a scoping review. *Physiotherapy Canada, 70* (2), 141–151.

Kleinveld-Middelkoop, M., & Peters, P. (2015). Patiënt, cliënt of klant? De zorgrelatie centraal. *Fysiopraxis*, 20–22.

Koes, B., Tulder, M., & Poos, M. (Zotero). *Hoe vaak komen nek- en rugklachten voor en hoeveel mensen sterven eraan? In: Volksgezondheid Toekomst Verkenning, Nationaal Kompas Volksgezondheid*. RIVM. http://www.nationaalkompas.nl/gezondheid-en-ziekte/ziekten-en-aandoeningen/bewegingsstelsel-en-bindweefsel/nek-en-rugklachten/omvang/#definition_2243

Kortleve, V. F. (2006). *De kracht van communicatie in de fysiotherapie*. Master's thesis.

Kortleve, V. F. (2015). Shared decision making: en shared approach. Over professionele fysiotherapeutische communicatie. *Physios, 3*, 29–35.

Lak, M., & Bijma, M. (2012). *Leefstijlcoaching: Kernvragen bij gedragsverandering*. Bohn Stafleu van Loghum.

Lakoff, G., & Johnson, M. (1980). Conceptual metaphor in everyday language. *The Journal of Philosophy, 77* (8), 453–486.

Lakoff, G., & Johnson, M. (2003). *Metaphors we live by* (1st ed). Chicago: University of Chicago Press.

Lang, F., Floyd, M. R., & Beine, K. L. (2000). Clues to patients' explanations and concerns about their illnesses: A call for active listening. *Archives of Family Medicine, 9* (3), 222.

Lang, G., & van der Molen, H. (1990). *Psychological communication: theories, roles and skills for counsellors*. Eleven International Publishing.

Latham, G. P., & Locke, E. A. (2007). New developments in and directions for goal-setting research. *European Psychologist, 12* (4), 290–300.

Lazarus, R. S. (1986). Puzzles in the study of daily hassles. In *development as action in context*. New York: Springer. 39–53.

Leventhal, H., Brissette, I., & Leventhal, E. A. (2003). The common-sense model of self-regulation of health and illness. *The Self-Regulation of Health and Illness Behaviour, 1*, 42–65.

Linn, A. J., van Dijk, L., Smit, E. G., Jansen, J., & van Weert, J. C. (2013). May you never forget what is worth remembering: The relation between recall of medical information and medication adherence in patients with inflammatory bowel disease. *Journal of Crohn's and Colitis, 7* (11), e543–e550.

Linton, S. J. (2000). A review of psychological risk factors in back and neck pain. *Spine, 25* (9), 1148–1156.

Lohmann, H., Siersma, V., & Olivarius, N. F. (2010). Fitness consultations in routine care of patients with type 2 diabetes in general practice: An 18-month non-randomised intervention study. *BMC Family Practice, 11* (1), 1.

London. (2020). Wikipedia. https://en.wikipedia.org/wiki/London

Louw, A., Diener, I., Butler, D. S., & Puentedura, E. J. (2011). The effect of neuroscience education on pain, disability, anxiety, and stress in chronic musculoskeletal pain. *Archives of Physical Medicine and Rehabilitation, 92* (12), 2041–2056.

Louw, A., Nijs, J., & Puentedura, E. J. (2017). A clinical perspective on a pain neuroscience education approach to manual therapy. *Journal of Manual & Manipulative Therapy, 25*(3), 160–168.

Louw, A., & Puentedura, E. (2013). *Therapeutic neuroscience education: Teaching patients about pain: A guide for clinicians*. International Spine and Pain Institute.

Lown, B. (1996). *The lost art of healing*. New York: Houghton Mifflin.

Lundahl, B., Moleni, T., Burke, B. L., Butters, R., Tollefson, D., Butler, C., & Rollnick, S. (2013). Motivational interviewing in medical care settings: A systematic review and meta-analysis of randomized controlled trials. *Patient Education and Counseling, 93* (2), 157–168.

Maes, J. (2007). *De hulpverlener—Tussen afstand en nabijheid*. KERZ vzw. Retrieved July 5, 2013. http://docplayer.nl/9954320-De-hulpverlener-tussen-afstand-en-nabijheid.html

Maher, C., Underwood, M., & Buchbinder, R. (2017). Non-specific low back pain. *The Lancet, 389* (10070), 736–747.

Maisto, S. A., Roos, C. R., O'Sickey, A. J., Kirouac, M., Connors, G. J., Tonigan, J. S., & Witkiewitz, K. (2015). The indirect effect of the therapeutic alliance and alcohol abstinence self-efficacy on alcohol use and alcohol-related problems in Project MATCH. *Alcoholism: Clinical and Experimental Research, 39* (3), 504–513.

Malani, P. N. (2010). The language of pain: Finding words, compassion, and relief. *JAMA, 303* (18), 1866–1866.

Mallen, C. D., Peat, G., Thomas, E., Dunn, K. M., & Croft, P. R. (2007). Prognostic factors for musculoskeletal pain in primary care: A systematic review. *British Journal of General Practice, 57* (541), 655–661.

Malliaras, P., Cook, J., Purdam, C., & Rio, E. (2015). Patellar tendinopathy: Clinical diagnosis, load management, and advice for challenging case presentations. *Journal of Orthopaedic & Sports Physical Therapy, 45* (11), 887–898.

Mann, K., Gordon, J., & MacLeod, A. (2009). Reflection and reflective practice in health professions education: A systematic review. *Advances in Health Sciences Education, 14* (4), 595.

Margalit, R. S., Roter, D., Dunevant, M. A., Larson, S., & Reis, S. (2006). Electronic medical record use and physician–patient communication: An observational study of Israeli primary care encounters. *Patient Education and Counseling, 61* (1), 134–141.

Marzano, R. J., & Kendall, J. S. (2006). *The new taxonomy of educational objectives.* Thousand Oaks, CA: Corwin Press.

Mauksch, L. B., Dugdale, D. C., Dodson, S., & Epstein, R. (2008). Relationship, communication, and efficiency in the medical encounter: Creating a clinical model from a literature review. *Archives of Internal Medicine, 168* (13), 1387–1395.

McLean, S. M., Burton, M., Bradley, L., & Littlewood, C. (2010). Interventions for enhancing adherence with physiotherapy: A systematic review. *Manual Therapy, 15* (6), 514–521.

McRae, M., & Hancock, M. J. (2017). Adults attending private physiotherapy practices seek diagnosis, pain relief, improved function, education and prevention: A survey. *Journal of Physiotherapy, 63* (4), 250–256.

Melin, J., Nordin, Å., Feldthusen, C., Danielsson, L. (2019). Goal-setting in physiotherapy: exploring a person-centered perspective. *Physiotherapy Theory and Practice,* 1–18.

Menendez, M. E., van Hoorn, B. T., Mackert, M., Donovan, E. E., Chen, N. C., & Ring, D. (2017). Patients with limited health literacy ask fewer questions during office visits with hand surgeons. *Clinical Orthopaedics and Related Research, 475* (5), 1291–1297.

Mercer, E., MacKay-Lyons, M., Conway, N., Flynn, J., & Mercer, C. (2008). Perceptions of outpatients regarding the attire of physiotherapists. *Physiotherapy Canada, 60* (4), 349–357.

Miller, W. R., & Rollnick, S. (2012). *Motivational interviewing: Helping people change.* New York: Guilford Press.

Morton, K., Beauchamp, M., Prothero, A., Joyce, L., Saunders, L., Spencer-Bowdage, S., Dancy, B., & Pedlar, C. (2015). The effectiveness of motivational interviewing for health behaviour change in primary care settings: A systematic review. *Health Psychology Review, 9* (2), 205–223.

Mosley, G. L., & Butler, D. S. (2017). *Explain pain supercharged.* NOI.

Munday, I., Kneebone, I., & Newton-John, T. (2019). The language of chronic pain. *Disability and Rehabilitation, 43* (3), 1–8.

Nijs, J. (2011). *Wilgen P van. Pijneducatie, een praktische handleiding voor (para) medici.* Bohn Stafleu van Loghum Houten.

Nijs, Jo, Torres-Cueco, R., van Wilgen, P., Lluch Girbés, E., Struyf, F., Roussel, N., van Oosterwijck, J., Daenen, L., Kuppens, K., & Vanderweeën, L. (2014). Applying modern pain neuroscience in clinical practice: Criteria for the classification of central sensitization pain. *Pain Physician, 17* (5), 447–457.

Noordman, J., Weert, J. van, Brink-Muinen, A., Dulmen, S. van, & Bensing, J. (2007). *Komt stress van de patiënt aan bod bij de huisarts?* https://www.nivel.nl/nl/publicatie/komt-stress-van-de-patient-aan-bod-bij-de-huisarts

Nova, C., Vegni, E., & Moja, E. A. (2005). The physician–patient–parent communication: A qualitative perspective on the child's contribution. *Patient Education and Counseling, 58* (3), 327–333.

O'Brien, T. (2019). Boreout, burnout and existential futility. *Vail 2019, 43,* 8.

Office of Disease Prevention and Health Promotion US Department of Health and Human Services. (2010). *National action plan to improve health literacy.* US Department of Health & Human Services.

Ogden, J. (2019). *Health Psychology, 6th ed.* New York: McGraw-Hill Education.

O'Hagan, F., Coutu, M., & Baril, R. (2013). A case of mistaken identity? The role of injury representations in chronic musculoskeletal pain. *Disability and Rehabilitation, 35* (18), 1552–1563.

O'Keeffe, M., Cullinane, P., Hurley, J., Leahy, I., Bunzli, S., O'Sullivan, P. B., & O'Sullivan, K. (2016). What influences patient-therapist interactions in musculoskeletal physical therapy? Qualitative systematic review and meta-synthesis. *Physical Therapy, 96* (5), 609–622.

Omgaan met mensen met een licht verstandelijke beperking. Voor verwijzers. (2014). http://www.meedemeentgroep.nl/media/med_view.asp?med_id=3190

Oostendorp, R. A. B., & Duquet, W. (2010). *Bio-psychociale manuele therapie: Hoe is het op de werkvloer?* NPI.

Orange, J. B., & Ryan, E. B. (2000). Alzheimer's disease and other dementias: Implications for physician communication. *Clinics in Geriatric Medicine, 16* (1), 153–173.

Oshima Lee, E., & Emanuel, E. J. (2013). Shared decision making to improve care and reduce costs. *New England Journal of Medicine, 368* (1), 6–8.

Østerås, B., Sigmundsson, H., & Haga, M. (2015). Perceived stress and musculoskeletal pain are prevalent and significantly associated in adolescents: An epidemiological cross-sectional study. *BMC Public Health, 15* (1), 1.

O'Sullivan, P. B., Caneiro, J., O'Keeffe, M., Smith, A., Dankaerts, W., Fersum, K., & O'Sullivan, K. (2018). Cognitive functional therapy: An integrated behavioral approach for the targeted management of disabling low back pain. *Physical Therapy, 98* (5), 408–423.

Owen, G., & Hunter, N. (2015). *Competency framework for physiotherapists working in occupational health.* Association of Chartered Physiotherapists in Occupational Health and Ergonomics. http://acpohe.csp.org.uk/publications/competency-framework-physiotherapists-working-occupational-health-ergonomics

Parreira, P., Maher, C. G., Steffens, D., Hancock, M. J., & Ferreira, M. L. (2018). Risk factors for low back pain and sciatica: An umbrella review. *The Spine Journal, 18* (9), 1715–1721.

Pauwels, R. A., Buist, A. S., Calverley, P. M., Jenkins, C. R., & Hurd, S. S. (2001). Global strategy for the diagnosis, management, and prevention of chronic obstructive pulmonary disease: NHLBI/WHO Global Initiative for Chronic Obstructive Lung Disease (GOLD) Workshop summary. *American Journal of Respiratory and Critical Care Medicine, 163* (5), 1256–1276.

Pel-Littel, R., & van Veenendaal, H. (2015). Gedeelde besluitvorming. *Bijblijven, 31* (8), 611–621.

Peper, E., Shumay, D. M., Moss, D., & Sztembis, R. (2013). The power of words, biofeedback, and somatic feedback to impact illness beliefs. *Somatics.* https://biofeedbackhealth.files.wordpress.com/2013/01/illness-beliefs-peper-shumay-moss-and-stzembis-2013-clean.pdf

Physiotherapy competencies for physiotherapy practice in New Zealand. (2009). The Physiotherapy Board of New Zealand. https://www.physioboard.org.nz/sites/default/files/PHYSIO_Competencies_09_for_web_0.pdf

Physiotherapy practice thresholds in Australia and Aotearoa New Zealand. (2015). Physiotherapy Board of Australia & Physiotherapy Board of New Zealand. https://physiocouncil.com.au/wp-content/uploads/2017/10/Physiotherapy-Board-Physiotherapy-practice-thresholds-in-Australia-and-Aotearoa-New-Zealand.pdf

Picha, K. J., & Howell, D. M. (2018). A model to increase rehabilitation adherence to home exercise programmes in patients with varying levels of self-efficacy. *Musculoskeletal Care, 16* (1), 233–237.

Pinto, R. Z., Ferreira, M. L., Oliveira, V. C., Franco, M. R., Adams, R., Maher, C. G., & Ferreira, P. H. (2012). Patient-centred communication is associated with positive therapeutic alliance: A systematic review. *Journal of Physiotherapy, 58* (2), 77–87.

Plack, M. M., & Greenberg, L. (2005). The reflective practitioner: Reaching for excellence in practice. *Pediatrics, 116* (6), 1546–1552.

Polaris, J. J., & Katz, J. N. (2014). "Appropriate" diagnostic testing: Supporting diagnostics with evidence-based medicine and shared decision making. *BMC Research Notes, 7* (1), 922.

Post, S. G. (2011). Compassionate care enhancement: Benefits and outcomes. *International Journal of Person-Centered Medicine, 1* (4), 808–813.

Pretorius, D., van Rooyen, M., & Reinbrech-Schütte, A. (2010). *Patient-centred communication and counselling: Principles and practice.* Pretoria: Juta.

Prioritising person-centred care: Enhancing experience. (2014). National Voices. http://www.nationalvoices.org.uk/sites/default/files/public/publications/enhancing_experience.pdf

Prioritising person-centred care: Improving information and understanding. (2014). National Voices. http://www.nationalvoices.org.uk/sites/default/files/public/publications/improving_information.pdf.

Prochaska, J. O., Norcross, J. C., & DiClemente, C. C. (2013). Applying the stages of change. *Psychotherapy in Australia, 19* (2), 10.

Ptacek, J., Ptacek, J. J., & Ellison, N. M. (2001). "I'm sorry to tell you..." Physicians' reports of breaking bad news. *Journal of Behavioral Medicine, 24* (2), 205–217.

Rajati, F., Sadeghi, M., Feizi, A., Sharifirad, G., Hasandokht, T., & Mostafavi, F. (2014). Self-efficacy strategies to improve exercise in patients with heart failure: A systematic review. *ARYA Atherosclerosis, 10* (6), 319.

Ramond-Roquin, A., Bouton, C., Bègue, C., Petit, A., Roquelaure, Y., & Huez, J.-F. (2015). Psychosocial risk factors, interventions, and comorbidity in patients with non-specific low back pain in primary care: Need for comprehensive and patient-centered care. *Frontiers in Medicine, 2*, 73.

Reynolds, P. M., Sanson-Fisher, R., Poole, A. D., Harker, J., & Byrne, M. J. (1981). Cancer and communication: Information-giving in an oncology clinic. *British Medical Journal (Clinical Research ed.), 282* (6274), 1449.

Ritter, A., Franz, M., Miltner, W. H., & Weiss, T. (2019). How words impact on pain. *Brain and Behavior, 9* (9), e01377.

Roberts, K. J., Revenson, T. A., Urken, M. L., Fleszar, S., Cipollina, R., Rowe, M. E., Dos Reis, L. L., & Lepore, S. J. (2016). Testing with feedback improves recall of information in informed consent: A proof of concept study. *Patient Education and Counseling, 99* (8), 1377–1381.

Rokeach, M. (1968). *Beliefs, attitudes and values: A theory of organization and change.* New York: Jossey Bass.

Royal College of Physicians and Surgeons of Canada: CanMEDS. (2006). *Royal College of Physicians and Surgeons of Canada.* http://www.royalcollege.ca/rcsite/canmeds-e

Rufa'i, A. A., Oyeyemi, A. Y., Oyeyemi, A. L., Usman Ali, M., & Bello, R. (2015). Physiotherapists' attire: Does it affect patients' comfort, confidence and overall patient-therapist relationship. *International Journal of Physiotherapy, 2* (5). https://doi.org/10.15621/ijphy/2015/v2i5/78219

Ryan, R. M., & Deci, E. L. (2000). Self-determination theory and the facilitation of intrinsic motivation, social development, and well-being. *American Psychologist, 55* (1), 68.

Saraiya, B., Arnold, R., & Tulsky, J. A. (2010). Communication skills for discussing treatment options when chemotherapy has failed. *The Cancer Journal, 16* (5), 521–523.

Sarason, I. G. (2013). *Social support: Theory, research and applications,* vol. 24. New York: Springer Science & Business Media.

Schaufeli, W. (2006). De psychologie van arbeid en gezondheid. *De psychologie van arbeid en gezondheid,* 1–22.

Schaufeli, W. B. (2018). Work engagement in Europe. *Organ Dyn 47.2,* 99–106.

Schönberger, M., Humle, F., & Teasdale, T. W. (2006). The development of the therapeutic working alliance, patients' awareness and their compliance during the process of brain injury rehabilitation. *Brain Injury, 20* (4), 445–454.

Scobbie, L., McLean, D., Dixon, D., Duncan, E., & Wyke, S. (2013). Implementing a framework for goal setting in community based stroke rehabilitation: A process evaluation. *BMC Health Services Research, 13* (1), 190.

Shachak, A., Hadas-Dayagi, M., Ziv, A., & Reis, S. (2009). Primary care physicians' use of an electronic medical record system: A cognitive task analysis. *Journal of General Internal Medicine, 24* (3), 341–348.

Shaw, A., Ibrahim, S., Reid, F., Ussher, M., & Rowlands, G. (2009). Patients' perspectives of the doctor–patient relationship and information giving across a range of literacy levels. *Patient Education and Counseling, 75* (1), 114–120.

Shay, L. A., & Lafata, J. E. (2014). Understanding patient perceptions of shared decision making. *Patient Education and Counseling, 96* (3), 295–301.

Sherer, M., Evans, C. C., Leverenz, J., Stouter, J., Irby Jr, J. W., Eun Lee, J., & Yablon, S. A. (2007). Therapeutic alliance in post-acute brain injury rehabilitation: Predictors of strength of alliance and impact of alliance on outcome. *Brain Injury, 21* (7), 663–672.

Sherman, K. A., & Koelmeyer, L. (2013). Psychosocial predictors of adherence to lymphedema risk minimization guidelines among women with breast cancer. *Psycho-Oncology, 22* (5), 1120–1126.

Siemonsma, P. C., Stuive, I., Roorda, L. D., Vollebregt, J. A., Walker, M. F., Lankhorst, G. J., & Lettinga, A. T. (2013). Cognitive treatment of illness perceptions in patients with chronic low back pain: A randomized controlled trial. *Physical Therapy, 93* (4), 435–448.

Sihvonen, R., Paavola, M., Malmivaara, A., Itälä, A., Joukainen, A., Nurmi, H., Kalske, J., & Järvinen, T. L. (2013). Arthroscopic partial meniscectomy versus sham surgery for a degenerative meniscal tear. *New England Journal of Medicine, 369* (26), 2515–2524.

Silverman, J., & Kinnersley, P. (2010). Doctors' non-verbal behaviour in consultations: Look at the patient before you look at the computer. *British Journal of General Practice, 60* (571), 76–78.

Silverman, J., Kurtz, S. M., & Draper, J. (1998). *Skills for communicating with patients.* Oxford: Radcliffe.

Silverman, J., Kurtz, S. M., & Draper, J. (2013). *Skills for communicating with patients.* Oxford: Radcliffe.

Slade, S. C., Molloy, E., & Keating, J. L. (2009). 'Listen to me, tell me': A qualitative study of partnership in care for people with non-specific chronic low back pain. *Clinical Rehabilitation, 23* (3), 270–280.

Staal, J., Hendriks, E., Heijmans, M., Kiers, H., Lutgers-Boomsma, A., Rutten, G., Van Tulder, M., Den Boer, J., Ostelo, R., & Custers, J. (2013). Dutch KNGF-guideline for low back pain. Amersfoort: De Gans.

Stacey, D., Bennett, C. L., Barry, M. J., Col, N. F., Eden, K. B., Holmes-Rovner, M., Llewellyn-Thomas, H., Lyddiatt, A., Légaré, F., & Thomson, R. (2011). Decision aids for people facing health treatment or screening decisions. *Cochrane Database of Systematic Review, 10* (10).

Statista. (2018). *Percentage of U.S. adults that frequently experienced stress as of 2017, by employment status.* Statista. https://www.statista.com/statistics/867030/us-adults-stress-experience-by-employment-status/

Staveren, R. van. (2010). *Patiëntgericht communiceren. Gids voor de medische praktijk.* Amsterdam: de Tijdstroom.

Stevens, A., Beurskens, A., Köke, A., & van der Weijden, T. (2013). The use of patient-specific measurement instruments in the process of goal-setting: A systematic review of available instruments and their feasibility. *Clinical Rehabilitation, 27* (11), 1005–1019.

Stevens, A., Beurskens, S., Köke, A., & van der Weijden, T. (2017). *Ready for goal setting? From a patient-specific instrument to an integrated method in physiotherapy.* Maastricht, Maastricht University. Narcis.nl

Stiggelbout, A., Pieterse, A., & de Haes, J. (2015). Shared decision making: Concepts, evidence, and practice. *Patient Education and Counseling, 98* (10), 1172–1179.

Strack, F., & Förster, J. (2011). *Social cognition: The basis of human interaction.* New York: Taylor & Francis.

Stubbe, D. E. (2016). The doublespeak dilemma: Effectively communicating with children and adolescents and their caregivers. *Focus, 14* (1), 60–63.

Suarez, M. (2011). Application of motivational interviewing to neuropsychology practice: A new frontier for evaluations and rehabilitation. In *The Little Black Book of Neuropsychology.* New York: Springer, 863–871

Sullivan, N., Hebron, C., & Vuoskoski, P. (2019). "Selling" chronic pain: Physiotherapists' lived experiences of communicating the diagnosis of chronic nonspecific lower back pain to their patients. *Physiotherapy Theory and Practice, 35*, 1–20.

Sullivan, W., & Developmental Disabilities Primary Care Initiative Co-editors. (2011). *Communicating effectively.* Health Care for Adults with Intellectual and Developmental Disabilities. Toolkit for Primary Care Providers. http://iddtoolkit.vkcsites.org/general-issues/communicating-effectively/

Talevski, J., Wong Shee, A., Rasmussen, B., Kemp, G., & Beauchamp, A. (2020). Teach-back: A systematic review of implementation and impacts. *PloS One, 15* (4), e0231350.

Taylor, S. E. (2009). *Health Psychology.* New York: McGraw-Hill Higher Education. https://books.google.nl/books?id=8b1fPgAACAAJ

Teal, C. R., & Street, R. L. (2009). Critical elements of culturally competent communication in the medical encounter: A review and model. *Social Science & Medicine, 68* (3), 533–543.

Testa, M., & Rossettini, G. (2016). Enhance placebo, avoid nocebo: How contextual factors affect physiotherapy outcomes. *Manual Therapy, 24*, 65–74.

Toolkit Laaggeletterheid LHV. (2015). LHV. http://lhv.artsennet.nl/web/file?uuid=13ece427-04f3-4c47-b63f-7546938b46b1&owner=90f6fa10-66c9-4bcb-a780-e442a27d18bf&contentid=107219

van Dulmen, A. (2012). Start communicating. *Inaugural Lecture. Nijmegen: Radboud University Nijmegen.*

van Dyk, N., Martoia, R., & O'Sullivan, K. (2019). First, do "nothing"… and listen. *British Journal of Sports Medicine, 53* (13), 796–797.

van Houdenhove, B. (2005). In W*ankel Evenwicht. Over stress, levensstijl en welvaartsziekten. Tielt: Lannoo.*

van Laarhoven, A. I., Vogelaar, M. L., Wilder-Smith, O. H., van Riel, P. L., van de Kerkhof, P. C., Kraaimaat, F. W., & Evers, A. W. (2011). Induction of nocebo and placebo effects on itch and pain by verbal suggestions. *Pain, 152* (7), 1486–1494.

van Wilgen, P., Beetsma, A., Neels, H., Roussel, N., & Nijs, J. (2014). Physical therapists should integrate illness perceptions in their assessment in patients with chronic musculoskeletal pain; a qualitative analysis. *Manual Therapy, 19* (3), 229–234.

van Zwieten, M., De Vroome, E., Mol, M., Mars, M., Koppes, L., & van den Bossche, S. (2014). *Nationale Enquête Arbeidsomstandigheden 2013. Methodologie en globale resultaten.* TNO.

Verberne, L., Barten, D., & Koppes, L. (2015). *Zorg door de fysiotherapeut—Top-10 gezondheidsproblemen (DCSPH).* NIVEL Zorgregistraties eerste lijn [internet]. www.nivel.nl/node/4677

Verheul, W., & Bensing, J. M. (2008). Het placebo-effect in de huisartsenpraktijk: communicatie als medicijn. *Bijblijven 24.2*, 38–44.

Vibe Fersum, K., O'Sullivan, P., Skouen, J., Smith, A., & Kvåle, A. (2013). Efficacy of classification-based cognitive functional therapy in patients with non-specific chronic low back pain: A randomized controlled trial. *European Journal of Pain, 17* (6), 916–928.

von Thun, F. S. (1981). Miteinander reden 1: Störungen und Klärungen. Allgemeine Psychologie der zwischenmenschlichen Kommunikation. *Rowohlt-TB, Reinbek bei Hamburg, Germany.*

Voogt, L.P. (2009). *De ervaringswereld van patiënten met chronische pijn.* Universiteit van Utrecht, Boom Lemma.

Vos, T., Flaxman, A. D., Naghavi, M., Lozano, R., Michaud, C., Ezzati, M., Shibuya, K., Salomon, J. A., Abdalla, S., & Aboyans, V. (2012). Years lived with disability (YLDs) for 1160 sequelae of 289 diseases and injuries 1990–2010: A systematic analysis for the Global Burden of Disease Study 2010. *The Lancet, 380* (9859), 2163–2196.

Vries, C. de, Hagenaars, L. H. A., Kiers, H., & Schmitt, M. (2014). *KNGF. Beroepsprofiel Fysiotherapeut.* KNGF.

Waddell, D., & Sohal, A. S. (1998). Resistance: A constructive tool for change management. *Management Decision, 36* (8), 543–548.

Waddell, G. (2004). *The back pain revolution.* New York: Elsevier Health Sciences.

Wahl, C., Gregoire, J.-P., Teo, K., Beaulieu, M., Labelle, S., Leduc, B., Cochrane, B., Lapointe, L., & Montague, T. (2005). Concordance, compliance and adherence in healthcare: Closing gaps and improving outcomes. *Healthcare Quarterly, 8* (1), 65–70.

Watson, J. A., Ryan, C. G., Cooper, L., Ellington, D., Whittle, R., Lavender, M., Dixon, J., Atkinson, G., Cooper, K., & Martin, D. J. (2019). Pain neuroscience education for adults with chronic musculoskeletal pain: A mixed-methods systematic review and meta-analysis. *The Journal of Pain. 20* (10), 1140.e1–1140.e22.

Weiland, A., van de Kraats, R. E., Blankenstein, A. H., van Saase, J. L., van der Molen, H. T., Bramer, W. M., van Dulmen, A. M., & Arends, L. R. (2012). Encounters between medical specialists and patients with medically unexplained physical symptoms; influences of communication on patient outcomes and use of health care: A literature overview. *Perspectives on Medical Education, 1* (4), 192–206.

Weinstein, N., Vansteenkiste, M., & Paulmann, S. (2020). Don't you say it that way! Experimental evidence that controlling voices elicit defiance. *Journal of Experimental Social Psychology, 88*, 103949.

WFD. (2020). *Who we are: Our mission, our values, our people.* World Federation of the Deaf. https://wfdeaf.org/who-we-are/

WHO. (2013). *Deafness and hearing loss.* World Health Organisation. https://www.who.int/health-topics/hearing-loss#tab=tab_1

Wijma, A. J., van Wilgen, C. P., Meeus, M., & Nijs, J. (2016). Clinical biopsychosocial physiotherapy assessment of patients with chronic pain: The first step in pain neuroscience education. *Physiotherapy Theory and Practice, 32* (5), 368–384.

Williams, K. N. (2006). Improving outcomes of nursing home interactions. *Research in Nursing & Health, 29* (2), 121–133.

Winkelstein, M. L., Huss, K., Butz, A., Eggleston, P., Vargas, P., & Rand, C. (2000). Factors associated with medication self administration in children with asthma. *Clinical Pediatrics, 39* (6), 337–345.

Wittchen, H.-U., & Jacobi, F. (2005). Size and burden of mental disorders in Europe: A critical review and appraisal of 27 studies. *European Neuropsychopharmacology, 15* (4), 357–376.

World Health Organization. (2013). *Health literacy: The solid facts.*

Yang, L., Manhas, D., Howard, A., & Olson, R. (2018). Patient-reported outcome use in oncology: A systematic review of the impact on patient-clinician communication. *Supportive Care in Cancer, 26* (1), 41–60.

Constraint-induced movement assignment: similar to the movement assignment but with restriction to the freedom of movement; the goal here is more precise and described in more detail.

Diagnostic process: the activities which lead to a diagnosis of the patient's health problem during the consultation – in physiotherapy this consists of the interview, taking the medical and patient history, as well as the physical examination.

Free movement assignment: similar to the movement assignment but now only specifying the final goal of the movement.

Movement assignment: the patient is presented with a movement action which they must try to tackle with the psychophysical possibilities available to them.

Movement description: the movement is now indicated in general terms. Formulation is given with regard to movement or combined movements, preferably in normal everyday language.

Movement regulation: this is usually and preferably applied in combination with an explanation of the movement. It consists of indicating the form of the movement along with details about the course, direction and speed.

Therapy process: the activities during the consultation which form part of the treatment for the patient's health problem, and which in physiotherapy usually consists of, for example, exercises, massage, manual interventions and information and advice.

Page numbers followed by 'f' indicate figures, 't' indicate tables, and 'b' indicate boxes.